CHOICES

CHOICES

The Life of an
Independent Woman

Jacqueline ClausWalker, Ph.D.

VANTAGE PRESS
New York

Published by Vantage Press, Inc.
419 Park Ave. South, New York, NY 10016

Manufactured in the United States of America
ISBN: 0-533-15187-2

Library of Congress Catalog Card No.: 2005901630

0 9 8 7 6 5 4 3 2 1

Contents

Acknowledgments   vii
List of Photographs   ix
Introduction   xi

I   A Woman from Paris   1
II   The Innocent Years   12
III   The Funny War   15
IV   Life in Paris During the German Occupation   20
V   The Departure of the German Occupation
        Personnel in August 1944   35
VI   The Life of a Female Pharmacist in the
        French Army   40
VII   Returning to Paris after the Nazi Occupation   61
VIII   America   64
IX   Tuoc in Vietnam: Nineteen Letters to
        Jacqueline and Suzanne   87
X   Nostalgia   119

Acknowledgments

Jacqueline thanks all the physicians and researchers she met during her years in the Paris hospitals, where she was an intern, for their teaching and devotion toward their patients, and their pioneering research. They are: Professor Ombredane, whose weekly patients presentations were very inspiring; Professor Fabre, the Dean of the Pharmacy School and Chief of the Pharmacy Department at Hopital Necker Enfants Malades; Dr. Weill-Hallé, who stubbornly fought for the use of the BCG vaccine to protect people from tuberculosis; Dr. Le Mee, who instigated new surgical approaches to Otorhinolargyngology with the help of Dr. Chevalier Jackson and the U.S., and a very special appreciation for the hematology teaching of Dr. Arnault Tzanck, the "father" of the science of blood transfusion.

She also thanks her friends and Simone's friends from medical school for their supportive friendship as they created an atmosphere of devotion to medicine and all its discoveries in the middle of the last century.

In the United States, Jacqueline thanks her teachers at the Union College of Pharmacy, the University of Houston, and Baylor College of Medicine. She especially thanks Dr. Roger Guillemin, the Nobel Prize winner, who helped her carry out her research for her Ph.D. thesis, and Dr. William Spencer, who gave her the chance to carry out research on patients with spinal cord injury.

She also thanks Dr. America Rodriguez (the daughter of Dr. Gladys Rodriguez) for her outstanding editorial review.

Finally, Jacqueline is most thankful for the help of her secretary, Betty Kilday, first during her publishing years at The Institute for Rehabilitation and Research, and now in compiling these memories so that they are readable by others besides herself!

List of Photographs

1. "Le Patron," Professeur Fabre, Dean of the
    Pharmacy School and Chief Pharmacist at the
    Hopital Necker Enfants Malades, 1940.   8
2. Professeur Weill-Halle, Chief of Pediatric
    Medicine at Hopital Necker Enfants Malades,
    1940.   11
3. Ambulance given to the Ear, Nose, and
    Laryngology Service to Dr. Le Mee, by the USA.
    From left to right: a nurse, a journalist, Professeur
    Le Mee, Jacqueline, and Dr. Tran Hu Tuoc, 1940.   16
4. Dr. Tran Hu Tuoc, 1942.   19
5. Jacqueline and Tuoc on the balcony of their
    apartment, rue du Theatre, in Paris, 1941.   23
6. Jacqueline in Paris, May, 1945.   43
7. Jacqueline and Louise in Berlin, winter 1945–46:
    ruins of the city.   53
8. Tempelhof, in Berlin. From left to right: a pilot,
    Jacqueline, a pilot, Bob and his fiancée, Louise (in
    front), 1945.   56

Introduction

Jacqueline's desire to write her memoirs was brought about by a question from her niece, Annie: "How did you manage during the war years to buy what you needed without any means of earning money, and having your family away and unreachable?" It was strange. Jacqueline never earned a living before the war. She had a small stipend as an intern, and her parents provided the rest of what she needed: a couple of summer outfits and a couple of winter skirts and sweaters. There were no expenses for outings, theater, or the cinema. When she needed or requested money, her parents provided it. Transportation was either by foot, or by buses or subways, which were very cheap.

Jacqueline lived in a modest apartment, situated on the right side of the Seine River. The family had no car and lived with few luxuries; her grandmother's motto was "life is a duty, not a pleasure." The room Jacqueline shared with her sister, Simone, held a small armoire for their clothes, and had no study space except for their beds. The family was nominally Jewish and attended synagogue only for weddings. Jacqueline was never taught any Jewish rites. Her Jewish school friends lived similarly.

Three generations of their forebears were French. Many died for the country and felt a strong allegiance to France. They were taught that working hard either intellectually or physically, was the moral way of life, and that women did not have to marry to survive . . . they only had to work.

They were also taught never to envy others, because they did not really know what others had, and to respect the other's beliefs—whether religious or social, as well as never to show off what they knew, to keep an open mind toward every human being, and never ever to feel superior!

To answer Annie, Jacqueline said: "A friend of the family, a chemist of deep Catholic faith, who worked at their grandfather's asphalt plant, was an idealist who had joined the French Resistance very early. He helped me by renting an apartment and often bringing cash, which with Tuoc's earnings enabled me to survive." There will be more about Tuoc later.

Another reason Jacqueline wanted to write the story of her life is that she was lucky enough, as a student, to meet and work with outstanding physicians who became part of the history of twentieth century medicine. Their idealism and constructive thinking had a strong influence on Jacqueline's constant desire to achieve what she was capable of.

The third reason is that Jacqueline's life during the Nazi occupation was typical of many French women who lived in Paris, Jewish or not, and is probably very similar to the life of many women in wartime or during any time that social values are disrupted.

Even at eighty-nine years of age, Jacqueline feels that a day when she does not write, paint, or take care of the garden . . . is sinful!

CHOICES

I

A Woman from Paris

In 1915, the First World War was raging throughout Europe. In December, in a small apartment of the sixteenth arrondissement in Paris, a baby girl was born to Suzanne and Gaston. Another girl, Simone, had been born eighteen months earlier. Suzanne was very disappointed that the baby was not a boy; she named her Jacqueline. The apartment was located on the second floor of a six-story stone building on rue des Vignes. The bedrooms, dining room and kitchen looked out over a courtyard and across to the kitchens of another building. There were only a few trees and bushes in the courtyard. The grand salon and the small salon faced a somewhat better looking old-fashioned private mansion with lovely gardens. The three bedrooms, the bathroom, and the lavatory were not heated and were very cold in winter.

Rue des Vignes was in the suburbs of Paris, near a park called the Bois de Boulogne and could be reached by a small train at a station called Passy. There were rooms for servants under the roof of the building, and a cellar where tenants kept coal, potatoes and wine. The cellar had no electricity and it was an adventure to go there with a small kerosene lamp. Because it was wartime, food was scarce, and the whole apartment was cold. Jacqueline was starving because Suzanne had no milk and all available substitutes gave her diarrhea; doctors said she would not make it. While Gaston was away, working for the army as an engineer, Suzanne decided to take both girls to the country to visit a bosom-buddy, Dino. Dino lived in Chabeuil, a small village on the river Drome, in the south of France, near Valence. Dino's architect husband, the only doctor in town, and the only Catholic priest, were all buddies. Good Doctor Arsac gave Jacqueline clotted milk (*lait caillé*). The entire medical faculty in Paris disapproved, but it was the miracle of miracles, and she started to improve.

The family finally returned to Paris where the big German guns (*la grosse Bertha*) were roaring night and day, and where life was still very difficult, with no heat and very little food. Upon receiving the medical advice, Suzanne went to the Zoological Gardens to collect donkey's milk for Jacqueline, because it was very similar to breast milk and digestible to newborns.

Finally, Jacqueline did well. Her first memory was being with her sister, Simone, in the lobby of the apartment building, drinking hot chocolate and holding a furry cat in her arms. On November 11, 1918, Germany signed a peace treaty. Suzanne and the servants went downtown to see the victory parade, leaving Simone and Jacqueline in the care of the concierge. The concierge's husband was a janitor at Jacqueline's grandfather's business, an asphalt and bitumen company with an office downtown and a plant north of Paris. The concierge's daughter was a secretary at the Perfumery Violet store, located at the Rue du Faubourg St. Honore. The president of the Perfumery Company was Suzanne's brother; so the concierge was completely trusted.

Memories of her younger years are not happy for Jacqueline. Madame Huyssman, whose son later became Minister of Education, taught the sisters at home. Their afternoons were spent walking in the Bois de Boulogne, where they were taken by the maid, Marie, in rain or snow. To avoid catching contagious diseases, they were not allowed to play with children they didn't know. There were gymnastics sessions, Greek dancing and ballet lessons, as well as piano lessons that did not last for Jacqueline, at the request of the teacher. Memories are filled with cold and boredom. The only fun times were Easter vacations when Suzanne took the family for two or three weeks to Chabeuil, where there was a garden, a tennis court, flowers, and fruit trees, but no electricity or running water. There were also summer vacations that took them away from the pollution of Paris, either in the mountains or at the seashore. Simone could not sleep at the seashore, so these vacations were usually in the mountains. Gaston was often on faraway exploration trips to find copper ore for mining, so the family was often accompanied by Marie, the maid who loved Jacqueline but was mean to Simone.

Finally the time came when the children had to attend a real school. Jacqueline had recovered from whooping cough, scarlet fever, upset stomach and other maladies. Colds and sinusitis often kept her in bed during the winter months. The effects of scarlet fever were the worst of all: the pain, the earaches, and the length of the illness, which led to Simone being sent away to her grandmother. Jacqueline remembers it being awful, but it was worse for Simone because her grandmother was mean to her! Jacqueline gave Suzanne a hard time because she didn't want to be away from Simone, who protected her, gave her some affection, and bolstered her self-confidence. The girls took the tests needed to enter school, the Lycée Moliere, in the same grade. Both passed, but since Jacqueline could cram for tests but was not intellectually capable of learning and remembering the contents of the courses, she fell to the bottom of her class. Simone, however, was on top in all subjects except art, which was one of the only classes where Jacqueline was the star! Jacqueline was also the star in the "old French" translations.

The lycée years were dull. Simone aimed for medical school, Jacqueline for a career in dress design and advertising.

She wanted to speak English and work in Paris and London, and had no other intellectual curiosity. In the thirties, girls were not admitted to the Ecole des Beaux Arts, where Jacqueline wanted to study, so she went to the Academy Julian, in the Latin Quarter. The school mostly trained women who wanted to teach art in the lycées. Jacqueline went through the curriculum in less time than the typical four years. Her only distraction was stopping each day for a couple of hours at the Grande Chaumière to sketch male and female nudes. She made no friends among the students, whom she found to be preoccupied with their looks and their dates.

Until 1939, Jacqueline lived with her family in the quiet apartment where she was born. She remembers the cold winters when she shared a room with Simone. The household consisted of their mother; her father, who was often away; a cook, Margot, who had a room in the attic; a maid, who slept in the apartment; and a cleaning woman. All the laundry was done in the kitchen and hung from the ceiling. The children's clothes were made at home. Jacqueline always felt like she was in jail because in addition to the servants, her family members employed the concierge's husband and daughter. Later, when she left the lycée, she began to use a public phone in a nearby café to avoid the listening ears at home.

Despite having a lifestyle that now seems lavish, the family actually had very little money. Jacqueline's grandparents were wealthy, but her father, even as a polytechnician with a degree in mining engineering, was unable to earn a living. This created a lot of tension in the family. At her grandparents' house, Jacqueline admired an extensive collection of impressionist paintings, Marjorelle furniture in the living room, a collection of antique Venetian vases and Chinese ivory carvings. She also admired precious little boxes in the informal parlor where her grandmother held court on Saturdays and all her friends dropped by for tea and cookies. But at home Jacqueline had nothing similar.

When they lived at home, young female students were sheltered from social and political news. Adults tried to ignore what was happening in Germany and Italy, and did not comment on the two dictators' aggressions. People around them feared international communism and revolution. There were usually no newspapers in Jacqueline and Simone's home when their father was away, and they had no radio! Suzanne spent most of her time with female friends, and Jacqueline and Simone were in the company of servants much of the time. The concept of anti-Semitism never entered their minds. The "Affaire Dreyfuss" was never discussed. Jacqueline became familiar with it only by reading *The Isle of the Penguins,* by Anatole France. Even when Jacqueline and Simone went to their respective professional schools, their tight schedule meant that they had little time or opportunity for discussions with other students. They left home at nine in the morning, and took public transportation. Everywhere they needed to go was accessible either by walking or using busses and the underground metro. After going to lectures, laboratories or studies, they were expected home long before dinner. They were allowed very few outings and spent most Saturdays studying. Sundays were spent eating and visiting at their grandparents. They were also expected at their grandparents' house for the celebration of the Seder and the New Year, where their grandmother read brief prayers.

When the family's financial status finally improved, they took summer vacations to Switzerland, Spain, and Italy. Some time around 1933, they spent a week in Venice, which was not yet filled with tourists. They even went to a lake resort in Austria, where they found there was already food rationing, in 1938! They did not think about what this might mean.

5

Jacqueline loved fashion. The girls' homemade garments were solid and indestructible, but inelegant. Later, they paid a small fee for their clothes to be made by dressmakers who worked in tiny dwellings. The garments they made were poorly cut but also impervious to destruction. When the girls became young women, their garments were made by the *couturières,* who copied highly fashionable clothing, had access to better fabrics, and were usually skilled. *Couturières* also worked in their apartments, and their clothes cost only a little more than the dressmaker's.

Jacqueline's grandmother chose haute couture, and also took Jacqueline to fashion shows. During her younger years, Jacqueline was usually poorly dressed, but she always wore round hats of various colors, and although she was nearsighted, she did not wear glasses, except at the movies or art shows. Glasses were not fashionable, so women went everywhere half blind.

During this period of her life, Jacqueline had two close friends from the lycée, Janette and Nicha. Both were top students. Their families met and liked each other. In these years, teenagers had very limited social lives—there were no outings and no dating! Simone was very secretive and did not share her private life with her sister—perhaps she had more social activities than Jacqueline!

During that time, Hitler was changing the face of Europe. Around 1934, the whole family, maternal grandparents and parents, told Jacqueline that art was no longer an option for her future. She either had to get married and start a family or go to a serious school that would guarantee her employment. They gave no explanation for the change! Medical school was Jacqueline's choice. This upset Simone who did not want her family to know about her many boyfriends. She became more and more secretive about her life. In contrast, Jacqueline was a chatterbox who blurted out every happening of her daily life.

Suzanne chose pharmacy school for Jacqueline. The first year was spent in a pharmacy accredited by the school. This pharmacy was located about two miles from the apartment where Jacqueline was born. She ran there, back and forth, four times daily. Meals out were unthinkable then! This was followed by four years of pharmacy school, at the University of Paris. She passed the course by completing several final examinations. If a female student were married, she would get her degree listed in her maiden name. Otherwise she could not practice! Jacqueline would eat lunch out, because her school was far from home, and she had to take a bus twice daily, or walk about three miles.

Prior to 1935, the field of therapeutics did not include sulfamides. Herbs, many of which are still being used in a purified and titrated form, were the only remedies, except for aspirin, Bayer's trade name for acetylsalicylic acid. Syphilis was treated with bismuth and mercury salts, and sleeping sickness was treated with arsenic, as it still is in poor countries. There were three hundred students at the pharmacy school lectures. Students learned about the composition of food, and the tests used to insure that the herbs were genuine. They were also taught biochemistry and the necessary laboratory skills to carry out a large variety of clinical tests on urine, blood, bone marrow and spinal fluid, as well as the tests used to detect poisons.

Jacqueline was so bored that she also attended evening lectures at a city hospital twice a week for a year, so she could become a pharmacy intern in one of the city hospitals in Paris. She passed a competitive examination, although her scores were at the bottom of the class. The internship lasted four years. Women were not made to feel welcome. The dean of the school, Mr. Fabre, was also the chief pharmacist at the hospital where Jacqueline attended evening lectures, and where she was able to complete her pharmacy internship. The hospital is called Necker Enfants Malades. It is located on rue de Vaugirard, and

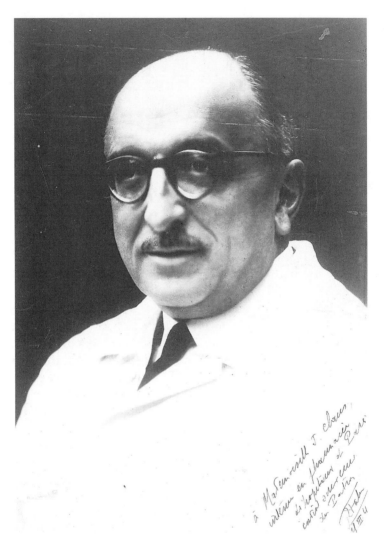

"Le Patron," Professeur Fabre, Dean of the Pharmacy School and Chief Pharmacist at the Hopital Necker Enfants Malades, 1940.

is very well-known. She worked there every morning until the start of the lectures, and every ten days she was on twenty-four-hour call and had to spend the night at the hospital.

Part of her work was preparing the drugs: pills, suppositories, injectables, etc. The other part, which she liked most, was to carry out, in a lengthy manner, all the currently available laboratory clinical tests. Early in the morning, the pharmacy interns had to do rounds with the physicians and their interns, and then suggest the available therapies for each patient. She was also trained in hematology, using single-lens microscopes. She learned to take bone marrow biopsies and identify their cellular patterns. She still remembers how proud she was when she identified a Nieman's Pick disease in a marrow sample, not realizing that this meant the young patient was soon to die.

During these years she met Aurora, a six-year-old girl who was orphaned during the Spanish Civil War, and saved by nuns, who cared for her in a Paris orphanage. While she was there, other children found out that she had a lump on her thigh. At the children's hospital it was diagnosed as a sarcoma. She was hospitalized at the Enfants Malades, where she learned French, and the whole personnel loved her. Sadly she could not be saved and was transferred to the Paris Cancer Hospital where she died a year later. At that time Jacqueline decided that research, not patients, would be her interest—there was too much pain in losing beloved patients. Another incident gave her some thought: one of her patients was a pretty, young woman who had an infection of the uterus due to an abortion done by an "angel maker," the name given to people who do illegal abortions using any available septic methods to do the fetal expulsion. The woman asked Jacqueline to help her get a job and after much coaxing, Jacqueline's grandmother hired her as a maid. After a few months of work, which were difficult because she had no skills and was basically lazy, the grandmother found her bleeding on the bathroom floor from another miscarriage! This was the end of Jacqueline's good deeds.

Jacqueline had some pleasurable experiences. She was very involved with the patients of Professor Weill Halle, who pioneered the Bacille Calmette Guerin (BCG) vaccination to prevent tuberculosis. The project was difficult because of the many deaths that occurred in Leipzig when hundreds of children were killed by an improperly prepared vaccine. Paris and all of France had many cases of tuberculosis, due to unsanitary living habits related to poverty. At that time there were no antibiotics. Even Jacqueline caught a primo infection of tuberculosis, which healed, but left calcified lung shadows that for a long time gave her problems when she took new jobs.

There were other pleasurable events. All the interns attended the outstanding Professor Ombredane's clinical lectures on sexual malformation in newborn babies. When Jacqueline later studied endocrinology she always remembered these lectures.

Jacqueline loved the laboratory work more than the drug manufacturing work. Hours were long, and weekends busy. She really enjoyed learning about the relationship between health, disease, drugs, and laboratory findings.

During this time Simone also went to medical school. She became engaged to a medical student, Georges. One winter, both girls had saved enough money to go skiing in a small village in the French Alps above the city of Grenoble called Mont Genevre. While skiing Simone met Jean. It was love at first sight. As soon as they returned, she broke her engagement with Georges. All was well until she became pregnant. She had an abortion which led to an infection. The whole affair was hushed up. She was treated with about twenty grams a day of Dagenan, the very first sulfamide developed in Germany. It saved her life but the abortion caused her problems having children later.

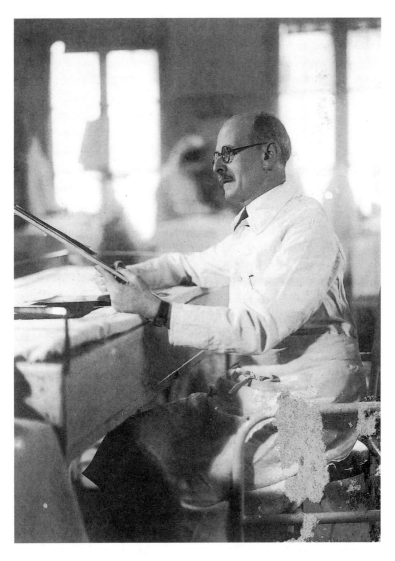

Professeur Weill-Halle, Chief of Pediatric Medicine at Hopital Necker Enfants Malades, 1940.

II

The Innocent Years

Under the influence of her friend Rosa, Jacqueline stopped being lazy and became a more serious student. Jacqueline had met Rosa in pharmacy school. They were matched alphabetically for the laboratory classes in which a group of four students worked around benches that had equipment for chemistry experiments. The two students spent all their school time together, even though Rosa married a medical student a few months after beginning their studies, and had a baby soon after. They stayed friends all their lives and had no other friends in the School of Pharmacy. Rosa was an ambitious, intellectually hungry, hard-working young woman, born in Kiev, Russia. She had had to adapt to a changing environment, money shortages, and life in several different countries. She was subject to racial and religious ostracism early in life, and became a very strong person.

There were other reasons for Jacqueline's positive change, including romances. The first was with Edmond, the cousin of Nicha, her lycée friend, whom she met briefly in Folkestone, England, while she was there one summer to learn English. Edmond lived in Guatemala. For several years they wrote to each other, but Edmond had to send the letters to Jacqueline's uncle, so her parents would not see them. Edmond came to Paris for French military training and to visit his relatives. When he left for Guatemala after a year, Jacqueline managed to meet him at his port of departure with the help of one of Dino's sons. She hurriedly returned following a night of marriage promises, but there was no mad love or sex—they were too brainwashed by their families for any behavior other than romantic. When Edmond returned, two or three years later, she met him in a café near the hospital where she worked, and found that his looks and personality appalled her. She had also just started another romance with a young, handsome and rich medical student, Claude DuFourmontel. She was fascinated by the fact that Claude was a member of the best sports and tennis club of Paris in the Bois de Boulogne, a place that she knew because her uncle was also a member. Claude had a sports car, his own apartment in a nice section of the city, and his own butler! Claude's father was a teacher at the medical school and a famous surgeon, the first to perform reconstructive surgery for the *gueules cassées*, translated "broken faces." These were injuries men sustained in World War I, which lasted from 1914 to 1918. Claude's father was rich from his work and his marriage to a wealthy woman. As is usual in the medical profession, he was surrounded by available females. He kept a mistress, so his money was not sufficient to put all three sons through medical school. Claude was the oldest boy.

For one year, after Jacqueline broke her engagement with Edmond, Claude called daily. He took her out on Saturday nights, and went with her to walk or ride at the alley of the Bois de Boulogne, where the "tout Paris" paraded their new clothes, new jewelry, new cars, new boyfriends or girlfriends, and new horses, on Sunday morning prior to the traditional family lunches. Claude also took Jacqueline to visit with the family of his previous girlfriend, Marianne, in their country summer home. Jacqueline was blinded by its luxury. It had tennis courts, valets, butlers, and gardeners. The relationship was acceptable to Jacqueline's parents because Jacqueline and

Marianne's grandmothers had been in school together! Then one Saturday, a year later, Claude's butler called to say "Monsieur Claude will not pick you up tomorrow morning." On Monday, Marianne called to announce her engagement to Claude! Jacqueline was stunned and mad—she was happy she was not in love with Claude.

Jacqueline's affairs motivated her to study and be ambitious. They marked a turning point in her life. Claude was attracted to Marianne for her money, and Jacqueline despised money—she thought. Later on, she befriended Marianne's sister and one of their nephews, and the friendships lasted all her life. Claude, however, could never face Jacqueline again. All of his friends from medical school, who were also friends with Simone, turned against him! Brilliant and dedicated, Claude Dufourmontel became "the father of plastic surgery." His brothers finally went to medical school but led unhappy lives. One of Claude's brothers tried to seduce Jacqueline at his other brother's wedding, but one Dufourmontel had been enough for her. The brother married and divorced, and Jacqueline met his ex-wife. She was a charming lady. Jacqueline's incentive to achieve was very strong after these romantic mishaps.

In 1939, a few weeks before the beginning of World War II, Jacqueline was annoyed that at twenty-four years of age, she was a virgin. She picked one of her sister's medical school friends to change that. The poor fellow was very surprised. He is now happily married and a grandfather.

III
The Funny War

In the summer of 1939, what the French called "the funny war," began, and interns were asked to live at the hospital. There was a shortage of medical workers because so many of the pharmacists and physicians had left for the war. Suzanne and Gaston had left Paris to take care of Suzanne's parents, who had moved to a small town near Vichy in order to avoid the vicissitudes they had suffered during the previous world war. Suzanne's two brothers were away with the French Army and could not help their parents. Simone had a commission to be a physician in a mental hospital in Blois, not far from Paris. All were without transportation except for the subway in Paris, some trains, their bicycles and their feet. Later, France was divided between occupied and free France. One could not travel from one zone to the other without special permission from the Germans. Jacqueline's parents and grandparents had settled in the free zone in a village called Neris les Bains, near Vichy. The mail was restricted to preprinted postcards. Of course there were no inter-zone telephones; radio broadcasts and newspapers were restricted to news censored by the Germans. Nevertheless, the resistance army was born soon after the beginning of the war and the German occupation, and somehow the British Broadcasting Radio (BBC) news could be heard.

In the hospital where Jacqueline worked, one of her bosses was Dr. Le Mee. He was an older man who had done some of

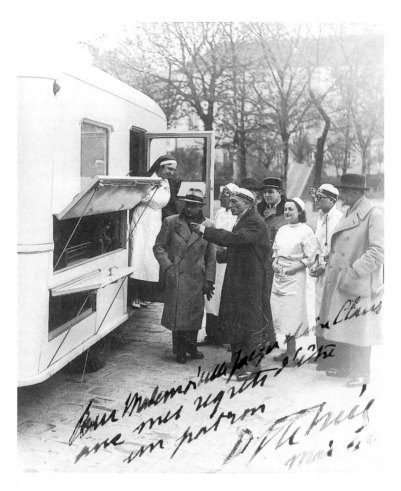

Ambulance given to the Ear, Nose and Laryngology Service to Dr. Le Mee, by the USA. From left to right: a nurse, a journalist, Professeur Le Mee, Jacqueline, and Dr. Tran Hu Tuoc, 1940.

his training in the USA with Dr. Chevalier Jackson, a pioneer in the ORL (Otorhinolargyngology) field of ear, nose and throat medicine. Jacqueline attracted Dr. Le Mee's attention and he wanted to take her out to dinner, but since he was a family man, he needed a social shield; he asked his assistant, a handsome Vietnamese surgeon named Tran Hu Tuoc, to join their party. It was love at first sight between Jacqueline and Tuoc. From that day on, they were inseparable. She left the pharmacists living and sleeping quarters, (salle de garde) located on the first floor of an ancient building, to eat with the medical interns in the salle de garde located on the floor above—which had never been done! Jacqueline was totally ostracized by the other interns in pharmacy. She helped Tuoc with mastoid bone surgeries, mostly by doing the light anesthesia by applying a mask delivering ether and air. Because of the shortages of nurses and physicians, she helped any place where she was needed.

In addition to her own hospital load, several times a week she pedaled to the Hospital St. Antoine, three to four mile bike ride, to work at the Hematology and Blood Transfusion Research Center, the first laboratory of its kind, headed by Dr. Arnauld Tzank and his colleagues. Many of twentieth century's hematologists were trained there. One of Jacqueline's projects was to examine, sketch and describe red blood cells in stored blood, to help to determine how long the blood could be used for transfusions. She was able to use a binocular microscope, which was wonderful. Another more routine project was determining the primary blood groups of numerous patients. At the time, transfusions were carried out arm to arm after blood samples of the donor and recipient were cross-matched. Such activities were curtailed when the Nazis occupied Paris because of the curfew and anti-Semitism. Dr. Arnauld Tzank was a Jew, as were many of his students. Nevertheless, most of them eventually became pioneers in hematology after their training in Dr. Tzank's research center, either in France or in other countries.

17

Throughout this period of Jacqueline's life, she was unconcerned with her clothing, usually wearing a long ecru blouse and a bibbed apron tied behind her back. Neither was bleached or ironed!

Her room in the very old building facing rue de Vaugirard was large, and the furniture was antique and drab except for the bed. She bought yards of chintz and recovered the chairs and bed, and made curtains. After this project, the other interns wanted to meet in her room! Even though it was at least two-hundred years old, the building had running water, which was probably added only a few years before. One had to cross a yard to go to another building to get to the showers. It probably is still the same! There was a bus stop, with a machine to take numbers to enter the bus, just below Jacqueline's window; she could hear it all night.

At that time Jacqueline was slender, with average looks. She was not much involved in female vanities, taking her profession very seriously! She was short, at five foot two and a half; and usually dressed in skirts, blouses and sweaters when she did not wear her hospital uniform. No one took notice of her as a rule. Tuoc was tall, extremely handsome, and was courted by all the female staff!

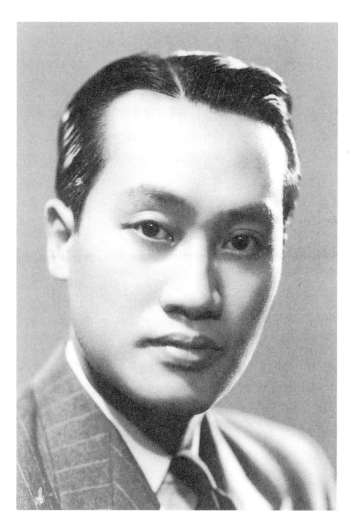

Dr. Tran Hu Tuoc, 1942.

IV
Life in Paris During the German Occupation

On June 14, 1940, the Germans invaded France, occupying Paris, and everything in the country changed. There was no mail or travel, and food and fuel were obtained only with special coupons. The day before the occupation of Paris, Jacqueline helped to organize group departures for people in the hospital who were scared and wanted to leave Paris, by helping to find funds and some food to sustain their southward exodus. Jacqueline was not afraid; she was very strong and efficient. There is currently a French film about the exodus called *"Le Depart"* (The Departure). On the day the German armies entered Paris, they lifted swastika flags wherever there were French flags; the most conspicuous was at the Eiffel Tower. They blackened the faces of all the clocks that were hanging as street signs at every jewelry store, because they showed the French, not the German, hour. They closed many streets to the French population. They established a curfew; no one could be out after nine at night unless they had a valid pass, or they would be shot. And after a few days, Parisians started to see lists glued to walls. These were the names of innocent people to be shot in retaliation for the killing of one German soldier or officer.

On the second day of the German occupation, Jacqueline was working in the hospital laboratory when a janitor came to tell her that a German officer was asking to see her. Very puzzled, she went to the hospital entrance—there was a young

German officer who introduced himself as a friend of Simone's, whom he met a few years before during a summer vacation in Austria. He went to meet Simone at the family apartment, rue des Vignes. Then he spoke with the concierge, who told him there was no one at the place, but maybe he could find out where Simone was by going to the hospital where Jacqueline worked. Jacqueline very coolly explained that under the new circumstances he should "get lost" and never return! She was very humiliated in front of all the anti-German pharmacy personnel. Throughout this period the weather in Paris was lovely, sunny and cool, making Paris very desirable to the German troops.

Three days after Paris was occupied by the Germans, Jacqueline arrived at the pharmacy to find there was a new intern, a Nazi collaborator. He told Jacqueline that she must leave the hospital and that if she ever came back in the pharmacy building he would immediately report to the Gestapo that she was Jewish—and that was the last moment of her internship! With some difficulty she rented an apartment on a nearby street, rue Blomet. It was on the sixth floor on top of an apartment building. It had a living room, a toilet and a kitchen, but no bathroom.

After only a few weeks, during which numerous Jews, communists, and gypsies were arrested by the Germans, there was a knock at Jacqueline's door at six in the morning. Tuoc was with her in the apartment. There was a commotion on the landing of another apartment across the hall, where two young violinists, husband and wife, lived. Jacqueline and Tuoc heard screams when the neighbors were taken away. They were never seen again. Jacqueline decided to "play possum" and did not answer the door. After a while, the men left and returned with the concierge, who said that Jacqueline was away on vacation and that the apartment was empty. The men left for good!

A while later the concierge came to Jacqueline's dwelling and told her it was safe to go, but that she had to leave immediately and without luggage, inconspicuously. Tuoc could stay and bring her belongings later. Tuoc was living in a nearby student hotel, so Jacqueline went there and stayed in his room. The wonderful concierge had saved Jacqueline's life. The concierge's sister, Madame Faidherbe, later worked for Suzanne and Gaston for many years, staying until her death. At this time Jacqueline made up her mind never to wear the yellow star, as the Germans had recently required the Jewish population to do.

As soon as the Germans occupied Paris, they took over all newspapers and radio broadcasting facilities, and broadcast only what they wanted the population to hear. Parisians lived in complete ignorance of what was happening in the rest of France and in the rest of the world.

Jacqueline's grandfather had a chemist, Mr. Herbos, who was working at his asphalt plant, and was in the French Resistance. After the missed encounter with the Gestapo, Jacqueline contacted Mr. Herbos, and he rented a very nice apartment for her under his name, on the rue du Theatre in Grenelle. Jacqueline stayed at Tuoc's hotel room for about a week. One night, very late, she was in bed with Tuoc when Gestapo agents made a search of the hotel, opening doors, looking at the people occupying the beds and deciding either to take them away for questioning or to leave them be! Luckily, they left. It was time to move out of the hotel!

When Jacqueline moved to the apartment on rue du Theatre, on the top floor of the building, there was nothing in the whole apartment but dirt. There were no electrical outlets, no stove, and no drapes or blinds. Then very unexpectedly, a woman rang the doorbell and introduced herself as Henriette Lechaux, and told Jacqueline that she brought all kinds of tools and would help to clean up and re-install what was needed. She had two young daughters, Jacqueline and Renée. Her husband was a colonel in the French army and was currently a prisoner of war. With her help, and the help of Tuoc and Mr. Herbos, the place was liveable within a few weeks. Jacqueline installed

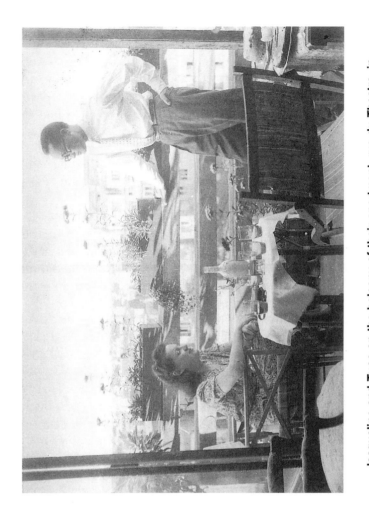

Jacqueline and Tuoc on the balcony of their apartment, rue du Theatre, in Paris, 1941.

roll-up shades for the compulsory black out. There was no central heating due to lack of fuel, and no working elevator because of the electrical restrictions, but there was a bathroom with an electrically heated water tank and a timer to heat the water during the night. Electricity was not restricted from nine at night until seven in the morning. What luck—this was easier than the rubber tub in the middle of the kitchen at rue Blomet.

For quite a while, life on rue du Theatre went smoothly. Many of the shop owners and their children had been patients in the hospital where Jacqueline spent four years, and even with all the shortages they were able to give Jacqueline and Tuoc packages with food or other necessary supplies.

During the funny war, Jacqueline was not worried about being away from her family because she was working almost around the clock, including weekends. Later, during the Nazi occupation, physical survival took a lot of time and energy—finding fuel, food, clothing, etc. She was so in love with Tuoc that being away from her family did not bother her. She had regular news about them from people who went to "free France." She knew her family was safe and together, and had more comfort than they would have had in Paris. She knew one uncle was in England and another a prisoner of war, but she was always an optimist and did not worry.

Jacqueline and Tuoc settled into the new place, even inviting friends for meager meals, and listening now and then to the BBC. A few months later, the concierge from Jacqueline's parents apartment called, in a panic, saying that because her family was Jewish, locks were to be put on the doors of their apartment, and all the contents would eventually be shipped to Germany. In a big hurry, Jacqueline and Tuoc located a two-wheel carriage owned by a man willing to take a load of furniture from Suzanne's apartment, 32 rue des Vignes, to rue du Theatre, which was about three to four miles. A lovely desk, a dressing table and some various items were recovered. The furniture eventually went to Stamford, Connecticut, to Simone's house. Very soon, many items which were not available in shops were for sale on the black market at high prices. Friends and relatives mailed packages from the country containing scarce items and food. These helped complete the meager diet that could be obtained, after long hours of waiting, with government-issued food coupons. Jacqueline was even lucky enough to get a telephone! Limited cooking gas was available for five hours scattered through the day. Cookbooks were published that were actually based on these restrictions. The limits were the same for electricity. Once Jacqueline used too much, the electricity was cut off for two months, meaning no hot bath and no light.

Madame Lechaux brought Jacqueline one bulb for the living room, by a long line ascending through the stairway. As the cold days began and there was no fireplace or central heating, a hole was cut in a window and a metal pipe inserted, going to a small coal heater in the center of the living room. It was very inefficient because the pipes were very narrow, and the coal was of poor quality. Several times Jacqueline took the subway to her grandfather's asphalt plant, to be given two bags of an oily charcoal. The small stove had to be kept going night and day to maintain even sparse heat. Matches and candles were not available, so the end of a long rubber line was inserted into a brass rod that had many holes. That was used to start the fire, with gas from the kitchen outlet. Sometimes Jacqueline got eggs from the country; these were kept in stoneware containers filled with rock salt, which was available, even though refined salt was not, and Parisians learned to refine the rock salt to use in food. Parisians also learned to make soap out of old grease and potash. Clothing was not available, so old clothes were mended. Soles made of carved wood were bought at the shoemaker and shoes were made out of odd leather or felt pieces. Old wool scarves were wound as headpieces to cover and protect the ears from the wind, rain, snow and sleet, mostly to be used while bicycling. Jacqueline also found old wool underwear from her father, who had used it on his exploration trips. She wore these items extensively, night and day.

One afternoon in 1941, Jacqueline received a telephone call in a café across the street. The owner called her to come to his café to get the phone call. She refused to go because she had a telephone in the apartment and all her friends knew the number. A few minutes later, two German officers and two French *milicians* (pro-Nazi civilians identified by an insignia on their lapels) were at her door with guns in their hands. They accused her of corresponding with the English as an excuse to search the apartment. They opened every drawer with their gun trained on Jacqueline's back the whole time. They stole some jewelry that had little value and some food, and went away very dissatisfied. Jacqueline immediately called a friend at the central police headquarters. She had met him numerous times while on night call at the hospital, where he was escorting patients for emergency treatments. Jacqueline had a very accurate description of the men, and later, both Frenchmen were arrested for multiple thefts. After their incarceration, she received small notes under the door, handwritten in slang, threatening retaliation! They came about every three to four weeks, until the end of the occupation. But the notes were not from the Gestapo! Her friend from the police headquarters told her that he was going to remove her file from the headquarters because the Gestapo could use it to arrest her for being Jewish.

In 1940, Jacqueline received news that her sister was getting married to Jean, who had been released from the French Army. Since the wedding was in Free France, she could not go. While Simone practiced medicine in the small town of Cavaillon, Jean could find work at a greengrocer's. Since there was a strong possibility that he would be shipped to Germany to work, one of his American relatives arranged for him and Simone to leave France. Jacqueline was able to obtain false papers and go to Free France to spend a few days with her parents, Jean and Simone. The ship Jean and Simone left on was one of the last to leave the French southern coast, in 1941 or 1942, and eventually reached Mexico City. They sold jewelry to pay for their passage. It took them another year to reach the U.S. They lived for a year near a copper mine in Santa Rosalia, southern California. Jacqueline had no knowledge of their adventures until the liberation of Paris. Strangely, she had no time to think about the separation. Survival took all the time and strength available.

So the lean years and the cold winters passed. Jacqueline had numerous head colds and tonsil infections but she couldn't check into a medical facility for help. When she needed a tonsillectomy, Tuoc operated on her at home. After the surgery she developed a mouth infection, called "trench mouth," which has a foul smell. This infection occurred in soldiers mouths during the First World War when they stayed in the trenches and had no way to clean their teeth. The infection was difficult to clear, and Jacqueline had gum problems for many years after!

Later that year, Jacqueline often became dizzy and nauseated, and felt miserable. Her friend Rosa's husband, Dr. Marc Labouré, sent an ambulance to pick her up in Paris. He sent her for rest and diagnosis to a clinic he used for his patients located in Choisy le Roi. The bed rest and warmth helped. The diagnosis was liver upset. After about a week she was sent home, where she realized that all her problems were caused by her being pregnant! Her periods were never regular, which made it harder to figure out her condition. She knew that as a Jew it was impossible to have a child because the minute the child was registered at the *mairie* district 16th, she and the newborn would be arrested and deported for being unregistered Jews, and the baby would be killed! At the same time, Rosa also became pregnant. Marc, her husband, knew she would have the same fate as Jacqueline since she was born a Russian Jew. He decided, as did Tuoc, that these babies should be aborted. Neither doctor helped—they made only rubber catheters available and refused to even discuss any other solution. Rosa and Jacqueline were on their own. Rosa's pregnancy was less than three months along, but Jacqueline's was more than four months. Jacqueline had a very difficult time with the do-it-yourself abortion. She had a lot of bleeding, but finally expelled the fetus, a boy already eight centimeters long! She put the tiny baby in a box and went to the Seine River, and with a very heavy heart, she drowned him. Tuoc did not go with her! He was a Buddhist and Jacqueline did not know the Buddhist philosophy on abortion but Tuoc was of no help, and it took her many months to recover, physically and mentally.

The years went on, and food became less and less available. Household gas was completely cut off. Old newspapers were rolled in small balls and saturated with burning alcohol—both of which were available here and there. Cooking was carried out on camping burners. There were brownish noodles, the green of carrots, rutabaga, and little else. In the street, people were wrapped in rags, walking in clogs with wooden soles and everyone was getting thinner. Children were short and thin, and were coughing most of the time.

When the Allied troops landed in Normandy, Parisians were full of hope! But about every other month, Jacqueline could still hear someone push paper under the door, and she retrieved threatening messages in slang. War news was circulated, mostly by word of mouth. Pin flags were placed on the Normandy maps and the U.S. Army's progress was followed daily! About five or six times, she received phone calls from friends and neighbors in the Resistance, and sometimes even German army personnel, warning that the Gestapo was on a rampage, rounding up Jews, Gypsies and foreigners to arrest.

These raids occurred for no apparent reason. Even so, men and women actively engaged in the Resistance were usually able to inform the population that mass arrests were about to occur. When warnings went out, Jacqueline went to Choisy le Roi, to stay with Rosa. Rosa was also threatened by the Gestapo. Her husband, a devout Catholic, was the physician at a Sisters of the Poor convent. These Sisters were ready to shelter those threatened with arrest, putting their lives and their convent at risk. Marc also risked his life, the lives of his two sons, and Rosa's life, by such unselfish behavior. In 2002, Marc was named in a ceremony in Cannes, among the few who helped others, as a sage. Rosa, now a widow, lives with her descendants in Cannes. Such underground resistance organizations saved Jacqueline from arrest, deportation and the horrors of the concentration camps.

Throughout all these terror-filled years, even with all the shortages of clothing and shoes, Rosa and Jacqueline managed to remain elegantly dressed. Women did not wear slacks then. They had dressmakers, hat shops and numerous black market sources, to maintain their Parisian vanities. Similarly, both Rosa and Jacqueline's escorts, Marc and Tuoc, were very vain and were clothed to perfection.

During these years, Jacqueline and Tuoc also had an enjoyable social life. They often bicycled to black market restaurants, and they took the subway to their destinations when the curfew was lifted a month or so after the occupation of Paris. One of their favorite places was a bistro on avenue de l'Opera, where Suzy Solidor was singing. Every now and then she stopped singing to welcome a group coming in, saying, "here comes a little subway." Then she resumed her melody! The subway, called Metro, rarely stopped functioning from early morning to very late at night throughout the German occupation. Many of the eating places sold black-market foods such as eggs or cheese, because most of them were able to get food supplies from the countryside. None of the restaurants they went to were heated, so they provided their clients with heated bricks to place under their feet. One time Dr. Le Mee invited Tuoc, Jacqueline and his head nurse, Madame Jendrau, to Maxims; when they arrived they found him seated with German officers. Jacqueline and Madame Jendrau apologized, went to the bathroom and left! Shortly afterward, Tuoc did the same. But that restaurant was heated!

Tuoc was often the physician on-call in various theaters in the city and he and Jacqueline pedaled there together. They had several close friends. Rosa and Marc lived in the suburb of Choisy le Roi. Marc had an electric car. Therefore he could bring himself and Rosa to the door of the underground Metro station, and could get together very often to enjoy the few restaurants still available in the city. Jacqueline and Tuoc were experts at sharing meals with their friends at home. The apartment had a very long living room, lined entirely with windows looking west toward the Eiffel Tower. The windows had to be totally blackened at night, by manually lowering rolls of tar paper! The windows opened to a large balcony, and in spring, Jacqueline and Tuoc often went to the flower market near the Isle of St. Louis to get soil and flowers to plant all along the balustrade of the balcony. This required many trips and a lot of stair climbing! The apartment was lovely, except during winter. It had no central heat, and there was a shortage of lights. They had furnished it with what they recovered from Suzanne's apartment and with a few pieces of furniture Rosa's parents had lent to them when they left for Mexico and had to empty their Paris apartment of all its furniture! Jacqueline's kitchen was small. She had a cleaning lady daily to do the dishes and the laundry, which was hung on a landing off the kitchen and often froze in winter. Many of their guests were Tuoc's friends, including an artist and painter, LePho, and his Parisian wife, Paulette, and another artist and painter, VuCao Dam, and his cheerful wife from Brittany. Often they had visits from a Vietnamese physician, Dr. Tin, from Amien, and his Danish wife, Inge. They also entertained their neighbors, Henriette Lechaux and her daughters, and a young couple who arrived in the building around 1941. When it was possible, they entertained Marc and Rosa, though they usually bicycled to Choisy le Roi to visit them. Their house was larger and had a garden, and their food supplies were better since they had family in the countryside sending packages.

Strangely enough, Jacqueline was never short of money, because it was delivered to her by Mr. Herbos, who was in the French Resistance. Members of her family in Free France provided the money. Tuoc was earning some money, but there were not many items available to buy. The utility bills were minuscule, and the rent was very low. Food packages from the country helped too! One summer, Tuoc, Jacqueline and Dr. Le Mee's secretary went to Brittany on the train, with their bicycles, and stayed in a hotel. The Germans were pumping the water to the hotel rooms! Access to the beaches was strictly prohibited because the German soldiers were building forts and training on horseback there. Tuoc and Jacqueline befriended a farmer's daughter who sold them eggs and butter. During the remaining war years, Jacqueline wrote to her pretending to be Tuoc, and the farmer's daughter kept mailing them food packages.

Jacqueline's sister and husband had left France in 1942, going first to Mexico, and then to southern California. Then a relative arranged for Jean and Simone to work at General Electric in Schenectady, New York, where they settled for a few years. Jacqueline had no news from them; her mother and father and grandparents were still in Free France at Neris les Bains. When her grandfather died in 1943, Jacqueline secured a false identity pass and was able to go by train to his burial. On the way back to Paris, she shared a compartment with two

German officers and a middle-aged couple. There was a lot of conversation between them, mostly about being against the Jews. The couple had a child, whose life was saved by Dr. Debré, a Jewish pediatrician whose family became well-known later. They argued hotly. The Germans made statements that they could always smell the Jews and detect them by their behavior. Jacqueline remained very quiet during the trip, and was very scared when she had to show her falsified authorization document as the train passed from free to occupied France. When she got off the train, one of the German officers asked her for a dinner date. She was happy that Tuoc was waiting for her at the station and refused the invitation for her! The Germans treated all Asians with courtesy because they assumed that they were Japanese allies.

Later that spring, the food supplies were reduced even more, so Jacqueline and her neighbor, Henriette Lechaux, decided to go to Amien, where Dr. Tin and his wife Inge had some food supplies. The weather was clear, and the bicycles were efficient. It was about sixty miles from Paris, and the two felt that they were going uphill all the way. When they arrived at the doctor's house, located near one of the springs that feeds the Seine, they were given champagne, and slept a few hours. The site was lovely and the water was clear. They fished and had a great time. The next day they left with heavily loaded baskets on their bikes. It was a hard ride, but after a few miles a trucker rescued them by putting them and their bikes on top of his load of flour sacks. When they were dropped off at one of the entrances to Paris, they were covered with flour, but very happy for the trucker's wonderful help, and very pleased to bring home some food.

By the spring of 1944, the American troops were very close to Paris. At six in the morning one day in July, about ten days before the liberation, Jacqueline heard banging on the door of the apartment. She did not open it, but asked who was there.

The answer was "the Gestapo. We are looking for Christine Claus, accused of corresponding with the British." Jacqueline responded that was not her name. They left, only to reappear on the balcony. There were four men: one German soldier, one Gestapo official and two French milicians, who were pro-Nazi civilians. The concierge had helped them by loaning a ladder! The men went through the apartment, searching all over, probably for money or jewelry. In the kitchen there was a box of cookies, a miracle that Jacqueline was able to prepare with one egg, a little flour and saccharine, during the very short evening-supply of gas. The men ate all the food! They didn't find much else, except for some nice gold jewelry which they took. Then they asked Jacqueline to get dressed to go to the police station. She decided on an outfit sturdy enough to wear in the dreaded weeks ahead. She had red lizard Richelieu shoes with thick rubber soles and a warm wine-colored wool suit, both of which she bought early in the occupation. She took her time, and was allowed to close the door of her bathroom. When she walked out, Henriette was waiting on the landing to find out where these men were taking her.

Within minutes, Tuoc had joined her at the apartment because Henriette had called him after hearing the brouhaha. They all went down the seven stories, but there was no Gestapo car at the entrance and the French milicians had left, saying they had other business to attend to. Jacqueline and the two Germans, who had not spoken to her in French, started walking toward the gardens of the Invalides. After a while they stopped and argued. Jacqueline felt like running off, but she was afraid of being gunned down, so she waited.

The German soldier left, then the Gestapo officer started to speak French to Jacqueline, telling her that she was nice, and that he would hate to bring her to the Gestapo, suggesting that if a little money could be given to his dispatcher, he would report that he was not able to find his prey! The Gestapo officer had a list of Jacqueline's friends who might be able to obtain some money for him. He suggested that they go to a café and use the telephone downstairs. So they sat at the terrace of the café, and Jacqueline was told to go downstairs to use the phone. Jacqueline called a few friends, and between Tuoc, Madame Lechaux and Madame Herbos, about six thousand francs were collected and given to the Gestapo officer, and the man disappeared. The whole time, the French police were watching helplessly, with no authority over German personnel, trying only to find out where Jacqueline would be taken.

She went back to the apartment, very shaken. These men, she thought, were not the Gestapo, because there was no Gestapo car at the door of the apartment building. They were ordinary crooks who needed money to buy themselves civilian outfits and disappear, so she decided it was safe to return to the apartment. Tuoc suggested that he should stay with her until Paris was liberated.

V

The Departure of the German Occupation Personnel in August 1944

Except for some more burning, bombing and shooting, nothing exceptional occurred in the vicinity of Jacqueline's Paris apartment until August 24th, 1944. No one knew if Paris was an open city or if there would be street fighting and destruction. Jacqueline was happy that after a few days of fighting and many deaths, Germany had enough love for Paris to make it an open city. It was only at the very last minute that the Nazi general, Von Sholtiz, made this official.

Much of what occurred in Paris has been described in the book and movie, *Is Paris Burning?* French television gave details on the sixtieth anniversary of the liberation, showing festivities and medals given in the rainy city.

At Jacqueline's place, a few days before August 24, 1944, Paris was very quiet; no police in the street. Then one day the city's walls were covered with posters promoting Charles de Gaulle, and others who supported the Communist Party. People walked around in the streets with tricolor bunches of flowers. Every now and then one could see a German car with protruding guns; there were also French cars loaded with FFI (Forces Francaise Interieures). When the cars met, their passengers fought. Then the city became very quiet again—and the barricades went up. Afterward, there was shooting all over town. In Jacqueline's part of town, Grenelle, rue du Theatre, rue de

Vaugirard, and rue de la Croix Nivert, there seemed to be a war among children, because the FFI were very young. A few German soldiers, called *les boches* by the French since the First World War, were hiding around town and on the roofs of apartment houses. The French *milicians* were getting into the shooting game also. One could hear the whistle of bullets night and day for twenty-four hours after the British BBC had proclaimed that Paris was liberated. The city was full of street barricades, which made it impossible to go anywhere, and trapped many Germans who were sheltering themselves in the Luxembourg Garden, in the Orsay Palace, in the military school and other places.

On the evening of August 21, a long summer day, Jacqueline and Tuoc took their bikes and pedaled toward the Porte d'Orleans, hoping to hail the liberating armies, but to no avail—there were barricades everywhere, so they returned to rue du Theatre. Around ten o'clock that evening, their neighbor Henriette called, saying that the army of General Leclerc was parading, but not go to outside because the city was dark, and full of traps and barricades. The next morning, Jacqueline and Tuoc went back to the Porte d'Orleans, where American tanks were passing through a delirious, enthusiastic crowd, but not five minutes had elapsed before guns started shooting from the Alesia Church. The crowd dispersed rapidly. The FFI, hidden behind the barricades, shot back with cannons and handguns. The noise was terrible—Jacqueline hung on to her bicycle under the porch of a house and watched the fighting. Tuoc was separated from her and very worried. About two hours later, she was able to bicycle back to rue du Theatre. Tuoc was already there—they were both nervous wrecks. The next morning, they walked to the Hospital Necker, where they could see the French flag go up on the Eiffel Tower, replacing the hated swastika. The rest of the day they watched the city fires from the roof of their own building. There were big battles to recover the military school and other fortified German strongholds. There was also fighting at the Porte de Saint Cloud where a huge cannon was fired incessantly.

The next morning, August 24th, they ventured outside to watch the Allied troops and tanks come in to a free Paris. During her walk, Jacqueline pinpointed a jeep with an American officer and went to give him a hug and ask him to join her and some friends to drink champagne.

At one-thirty that afternoon, without even thinking about lunch, Jacqueline and Tuoc went with Henriette and her daughters to go see the Leclerc Army and General DeGaulle parade down the Champs Elysees. They found a good location near the sidewalk, under a burning sun. They had already watched General de Gaulle on foot, near the Rond Point des Champs Elysees, but when he reached the Place de la Concorde, fighting started again with bullets fired by FFI, milicians and Germans. The trip home involved lying on their bellies, seeking the shelter of walls, in order not to be shot. They finally reached rue du Theatre, only to encounter FFI firing from rooftops. Hoping to find shelter at home, they climbed the seven stories, only to face more FFI firing from the building across the street. Jacqueline ran downstairs, crossed the street, and asked the first FFI person she met what was going on—she was told that there was firing from the roof of her apartment. The FFI fellow went up, checked Jacqueline's apartment and roof, and left, saying that everything was all right. A short while later, Jacqueline was in the bathroom taking a cold shower because the weather was so hot, when she heard a lot of noise and saw plaster over the bathtub disintegrating. She grabbed a towel and went into the living room and saw Tuoc on the floor. She felt wind on her neck and saw the wall plaster crumble! It was a bullet! Dressed in only a towel, she crawled on the floor and then ran downstairs to bring the FFI group back. They did not understand what was going on and believed that Tuoc had been shooting at them. They asked Jacqueline and Tuoc to sit down so they could again inspect the place. One of the FFI men was a little smarter than the rest; he finally understood that someone was shooting at Tuoc and Jacqueline and that the shooting was *at* the apartment and not *from* the apartment. A great mix-up had occurred because of crossed signals; the FFI fighters saw people in the house across the street, which was Jacqueline's apartment. They thought they were enemies and shot at them. The result was two bullets lodged in the inside wall and two more outside. The roofs of Paris are very accessible, leading from building to building. Many are partially flat and have small attic windows, making it easy to get in and out and from one building to another. The rest of the day, after so much turmoil, Tuoc and Jacqueline were exhausted. She went out to return her bike to the garage and saw the American officer she had talked to at the parade, in a jeep parked at the door. He was accompanied by two friends. Everyone climbed the seven flights of stairs, including Henriette and her daughters, to drink champagne. All evening one could hear the bells of Notre Dame ringing! The Americans were very pleased. They were news photographers who left Paris the following day to follow the armies.

After these events, Jacqueline and Tuoc were too tired to think about dinner. They tried to stay awake all night to see if someone was still on the roof, friend or foe! They were ready to rest, but at dawn the Germans started shooting bombs over the city, from many low-flying airplanes, burning La Halle aux Vins, and leaving great clouds of smoke. There was an air-raid alert, so Jacqueline and Tuoc and the neighbors went into the shelter in the cellar. Jacqueline was dressed up to go out, and the stairway and the cellar were completely in the dark. After a while, they tried to return to their respective dwellings, but had to return to the cellar because there was another alert.

They all felt wonderful, despite their adventures, because although the war was not yet over, it was the end of the German occupation of Paris.

VI

The Life of a Female Pharmacist in the French Army

Part One: The Paris Year

Although Paris had been liberated on August 24, 1944, the war was not over. The lack of heat and food was still acute. Finally, Jacqueline's family, her grandmother and her parents returned to Paris. They had nothing, no place to stay, and no belongings. They had to start over. They stayed a few days in Jacqueline's apartment, but since there was only one bedroom, it was very cramped. Suzanne's cousin, Germaine, who had been in the Resistance, had bought several apartments in a building on rue Scheffer, and she offered one to Suzanne and Gaston to rent. The small apartment, close to the Place du Trocadero, had only one bedroom and one bathroom.

After several months, Suzanne's brother, who had enrolled in the British Army after leaving France at Dunkerque, came back to Paris and was able to recover his apartment that had been occupied by the Germans because he fought in both world wars. It was large enough for him and his mother. Suzanne's other brother had been a prisoner of war. Because he had fought in the 1914–1918 war, he was repatriated to France. Around 1941 he had joined the French Resistance and was arrested by the Gestapo. He was deported and was lost somewhere in Lithuania. His disappearance was never documented.

Many other family members and friends could not be found, even years later.

Because peace had returned, and Jacqueline's family was in Paris, Tuoc thought that it was time to get married. Jacqueline panicked—she did not want to settle down yet! So at the end of 1944 she joined the AFATS (Auxiliary Femelle Armée de Terre) as a lieutenant pharmacist. The women who volunteered were examined for fitness at the military school situated in the Invalides military compound, in the same manner as the men. Their height, the condition of their teeth, and their chest measurements were recorded. Since the women were not submitted to tests for venereal diseases, many prostitutes, infected with gonorrhea or syphilis were able to join the female army. One of the first things the medical women organized was an all-female hospital, Hopital Inkerman, located in Neuilly on Boulevard Inkerman. Before being accepted in the AFATS, all newcomers were checked for contagious diseases, including tuberculosis, gonorrhea and syphilis.

Shortly after volunteering, Jacqueline met Louise, a young female physician from Brittany, who was liberated by the American army from a prison in Fresnes, located in the outskirts of Paris. She had been imprisoned six months after being arrested as a member of the French Resistance and had been held in a cell with General de Gaulle's sister. Jacqueline thought that perhaps if Louise shared her apartment she could slowly detach herself from Tuoc by always being in the company of her roommate, thus making intimacy impossible. The main reason Tuoc insisted on getting married was that he was offered a position to take over the Dr. Le Mee's medical practice, which meant instant success and money. Tuoc generously offered to share the wealth with Jacqueline, thereby renouncing his lifelong dream of returning to communist Vietnam, practicing his medical and surgical skills, and helping his compatriots by building up medical facilities and organizing a health department. Jacqueline felt blackmailed. Suzanne and Gaston were very fond of Tuoc and wanted her to accept and become Tuoc's wife, which made it even more difficult for her to say no.

Around this time, Jacqueline and Louise joined the Red Cross volunteers with a group of other affluent Parisian women who spoke English and were socially able to entertain. They were hostesses for the Red Cross in various elegant hotels and restaurants, as well as in their homes. The social contacts with U.S. officers allowed both women to improve their English. In addition, Louise and Jacqueline met two young Signal Corps lieutenants at a friend's party for U. S. officers, and became very friendly with them. One was from Alabama, and married Louise much later. The other returned to his American sweetheart, married and had many children, but sadly lost his wife. A few years later he asked Jacqueline to marry him and take over the care of his many children! When these American officers were in Paris, they did a lot of sight-seeing with the women. These outings gave Jacqueline and Louise a chance to enjoy dancing and good food, often at the Hotel Crillon, and to learn to enjoy American music and improve their Americanized English.

Throughout that year both women were bicycling to the Hopital Inkerman to carry out their professional duties. It was a very long ride from Grenelle to Neuilly!

After being at the local women's hospital for a year, an opportunity arose for Jacqueline and Louise to join the occupation troops as a pharmacist and doctor in Berlin. Both thought it would be morally fulfilling and patriotic to sign up for these positions. Jacqueline also felt that getting away was perhaps the only way to decide what to do with her life. So they signed up to join a French military hospital situated in the French occupation zone in northern Berlin. The Russian, British, and the American armies also occupied Berlin in four geographical zones.

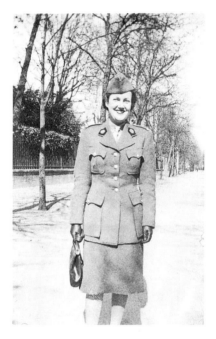

Jacqueline in Paris, May, 1945.

Part Two: A Furlough from the French Medical Corps

Before leaving for Germany, French officers were allowed to take a week's furlough. Louise and Jacqueline's destination choice was Cannes, on the French Riviera. September weather in Cannes is heavenly—warm and dry. They left Paris on a slow, crowded train, and after many hours without food or water or overnight accommodations, arrived in Marseilles. As they were leaving the train station they asked where they could go to eat, but found that there were no places for civilians or for army people. It was the end of the day, so they gave up on food and tried to find a room for the night. None were available, except by the hour. Since they were on foot and did not know the city, they could not go very far from the railway station. Discouraged, they returned to the train station to settle in for the night in their train compartment, which was parked for the night in the station! They drank some water after locating a potable water spigot. They wanted to eat a can of sardines that was in their luggage, but had no can opener. They had to ask a passing French soldier to help them open the can of sardines, which he did with great difficulty, having only a knife available. Mosquitoes were aggressive and numerous, and after a miserable night, they couldn't even think of breakfast. The train for Cannes was leaving at midday, so they had time to venture out again in Marseilles.

The town was full of American army personnel. Louise and Jacqueline thought since they were in uniform they could seek help from an American officer in locating a place to eat—and it worked. Since no French facility was available, they were taken to a U.S. Army mess hall, told to wait outside, and given a coca cola and fried chicken to eat out in the street! Both items were totally new to Louise and Jacqueline; the servings were enormous and the food tasted delicious. By the end of the day they had reached Cannes. They walked to the Hotel Carlton where they had a room for a week. The Hotel Carlton is the most luxurious hotel in Cannes, but in September, 1945, there was no service or hot water, and the lukewarm tap water was not drinkable. "Do not drink" signs were everywhere. In other words, the French Medical Corps had a hotel for their personnel for sleeping only, with no food or water, or ablution!

In 1945, Cannes was a very small town with few winter residents, frequented mostly by tourists. The main thoroughfare, La Croisette, was a large, beautifully landscaped avenue along the waterfront, dominated by cliffs and uphill streets. In addition to the high luxury hotels built for tourists at the turn of the twentieth century, there were numerous villas and palaces surrounded by landscaped gardens. Some were along the city-side of the street, some on rocky promontories over the Mediterranean Sea. Many of the cliffs have vertical walls deep in the sea, forming natural swimming holes. Just east of Cannes there is a hotel, Cap d'Antibes, built on a rocky promontory, Eden Rock, that has several of these pools and is embellished artistically to make space for lounge chairs, bars and diving boards. Cap d'Antibes Hotel is still there. In 1945, the U.S. military occupied all of the hotels where they had officers' clubs offering luxury dining, alcohol, music, orchestras and dancing. The older part of the city, located west on a cliff over a commercial airport, is not very interesting historically. There was only one commercial street, called rue d'Antibe, joining the tourist section of the city to the old section. The *palais* of the film festival did not exist then. It is now located at the west end of the Croisette. There was one casino, also along the Croisette. At that time all of Cannes could be explored by walking. Antibes was further and could only by reached by car, boat, or train. There was, and there is still is, a train stop at every small coastal city.

Jacqueline and Louise discovered the American Red Cross mess hall located on the Croisette over the beach, where they could drink weak coffee and eat as many doughnuts as they wanted without paying. Then they decided to fraternize. They met a pretty French girl, Mamie Arene, who was also a lieutenant in the French Army, and whose father was a general and a physician in the French Army. Mamie had a car and a chauffeur, who shared her bed. She was generous, and with her car driven by the chauffeur, Jacqueline and Louise went everywhere on the coast, managing to be invited to many officer's clubs, where they ate luxurious food and had occasional romances.

Along the way Jacqueline made a mistake. On the terrace of a café on the waterfront, she befriended an older military man from the French Legion While they were sitting at a table he grabbed her, took her by force to his dwelling in a narrow alley of the old city of Cannes overlooking the port, locked the door and screamed out his hatred for all females and all Americans. He put the door key in his pocket, and then he went to his bed, still grabbing Jacqueline. Luckily he was very drunk and within minutes he was asleep. Listening to his frequent snores, she dug through his pocket for the key, silently opened the door, and ran the two miles back to the hotel where Louise was frantically waiting for her, ready to call the police.

She made another mistake because of her ego. Both girls went to the Hotel Cap d'Antibes, and sat on the edge of one of the many natural pools, which are part of the beach and carved into the rock. This one had a very high diving board for jumping into deep water. Another French military woman climbed up the diving ladder, looked at the deep water and then climbed down. Jacqueline thought this was a humiliating way for a French military officer to act, so she climbed up, closed her eyes and jumped from the highest platform. It took a very long time to reach the water. She never dove again! After exchanging addresses with many U.S. officers and enjoying a wonderful vacation, the women returned to Paris to start their trip to Berlin. They had enjoyed the sun, the sea, good food, and a freedom that neither had ever experienced before!

Part Three: The Berlin Year

Jacqueline and Louise's friendship was very strong. Many of the American men asked them if they were involved with each other. At that time, homosexuality was not in fashion, and not being very knowledgeable about it, they were appalled!

Jacqueline's vanity concerning clothing was forever present. Their uniforms were British-made. They consisted of Eisenhower jackets, straight wool skirts, khaki cotton shirts, and neckties. Even their long underwear and silk stockings were khaki! As medical personnel, they were Second Lieutenants in the French Army Medical Corps. Pharmacists had green insignias and physicians had red ones for the lapels of their jackets. They had slacks, in addition to their skirts. Before leaving for Germany, both Louise and Jacqueline had uniforms custom-made by a French tailor specializing in military uniforms, which had a better fit! Once in the army, women had to renounce being fashionable, though the custom-made uniforms had some character.

On a dreary day in mid-November, 1945, Louise and Jacqueline, wearing their khaki sub-lieutenant uniforms with slacks, were ready to leave for Berlin. They had packed one large army trunk for both of them and carried a small bag of khaki canvas, called a "musette" by the French Army. These bags contained a change of underwear, eating utensils and little else. Wearing their slacks made them more comfortable for the trip. The shoes were not very good quality. The silk khaki underwear was provided by the British, as were the short jacket and high-necked shirt. Their outerwear, called "capote" was made of very heavy wool, and it was so stiff it could stand by itself on the floor. These were leftover French war supplies from the two world wars. For their heads, they had the usual kepi. All of this was somewhat water-repellant and very unattractive.

Following their travel orders, Louise and Jacqueline and their trunk reached the Gare du Nord in an army vehicle, which was sent to their Paris apartment. The two women traveled by train for many hours in a cold compartment with no access to food or drinks. They sat on benches in a very crowded train where all the other passengers were men. Finally the train stopped in the country in the middle of nowhere, in a field where army trucks were waiting for the traveling soldiers. All the passengers were taken to an army depot in the vicinity of Strasbourg and dumped without any directions. Jacqueline and Louise examined their orders. They had to meet their group in Strasbourg in a specific building, but they had no idea how to get there. General Lechaux, the husband of their neighbor, Henriette, had been liberated from prison camp and was stationed in Strasbourg. Fortunately they had his phone number, and called him. He suggested that he meet them at his headquarters, and from there he could help them! They were told to just leave the trunk (*la cantine*) with adequate address labels.

Louise and Jacqueline went to a highway and hitchhiked, as there was no other transportation available. The vehicle that stopped was a truck loaded with coal, so they climbed up on top of the coal and arrived at his headquarters very black and dirty! They arrived about twenty hours since their departure from the railroad station in Paris. General Lechaux, the dear man, managed to help them get cleaned up and fed. Then they joined their convoy going to Berlin. The weather was dreary, cold and wet, and the pre-war cars of the convoy, about twenty of them, were in sorry mechanical condition. Their drivers were very young and inexperienced; they had no previous driving experience except for the driving lessons to get their licenses. Nobody in France had had cars available for four to five years during the German occupation.

Jacqueline and Louise and all the others were given very small food rations to carry along, and the convoy started towards its destination. After dark, the convoy stopped near a forest for them to spend the night. There was no hot food or drink available, and the members of the convoy were told to sleep in the cars! Jacqueline and Louise were both fluent in English, and a soldier had told them that there was a camp of black American GI's nearby, so they set out on foot toward the camp, hoping for some hot coffee and a friendly welcome! They did not know that at that time, black and white people did not mix socially in America. Regardless, some of the black soldiers were very kind and gave them hot coffee; then they quickly returned to their night quarters in the unheated cars. Early in the morning the convoy left for Baden Baden, where they were assigned a hotel room, without heat or hot water. Luckily they found a cake of soap in the musette and were able to clean up with cold water, after which there was enough daylight to take a walk in the forest. Then they went to the eating quarters where a meager meal was served to small groups, one at a time, because flatware and dishes were scarce and had to be washed after each group ate. The women had tin mugs in the musette, so they were served sooner. There was plenty of wine as usual. Jacqueline never had any desire to visit Baden Baden since!

The following day was cold and rainy; at eight in the morning they were back in their assigned car. They rode miles on small roads, since many of the best roads were unusable due to Allied forces bombings. After a few hours, their car had a flat tire but there were no tools for repair. Luckily, a passing car from the Swiss Red Cross stopped and its passengers helped the driver change the tire. Before leaving, the convoy gave all the French soldiers strong alcohol to drink and warm up. Late in the day the convoy reached an industrial town that was in ruins. Each member of the convoy was given a *billet de logement*, a special letter that was needed to obtain lodging at local dwellings. Louise and Jacqueline started out on foot under a misty rain and stopped at the address given in their billet. The lodging was a dingy building where a man grudgingly showed them a room in an apartment located on a third floor, opening to a landing with many apartments. The landing had one toilet for all the tenants. The toilet was open to the wind and the rain! There was no heat and no bath, so they went to sleep with their clothes on, and with empty bellies. Jacqueline and Louise had to use the toilet but didn't want to venture out. A big black leather boot was the next best thing!

Departure was planned for early morning, but many of the cars in the convoy were stalled. By midday there were only a few cars left; the others were either gone or being repaired. After leaving in what remained of the convoy, the driver stopped in a very small village where Jacqueline had an unexpected mishap: the zipper of her slacks broke. "No problem," said one soldier. "We will take you to the tailor shop." But the tailor had no zipper. First he gave Jacqueline a blanket to wrap around herself, and because there was no other space, he asked her to wait in the display window of the shop. Every passerby looked in! When the tailor returned the slacks with a seam to replace the zipper, Jacqueline had to show him that there was no way to put on the garment. After a long search, the tailor located one button and made a buttonhole, and the problem was resolved . . . at no cost!

At the end of the short winter day, the convoy's next stop was a farmhouse. Their unhappy German hosts treated them correctly but were unfriendly. Jacqueline, Louise and the French soldiers had hot food, and slept in their own rooms with wonderful feather beds. The houses had some heat and facilities for minor ablutions. In the morning, the women heard a lot of banging outside, and when they looked out the window they saw the drivers attempting to start the few vehicles that were still with the convoy. But their car could not be started even after two or three hours of trying, so Jacqueline and Louise packed their meager belongings and left by foot toward an autobahn (freeway) that was supposedly not far away. The first American jeep drivers that stopped were very friendly, but could not take them to Berlin. They offered to help any way they could, so Louise and Jacqueline asked if they could find a place for the women to have a warm shower. The drivers took them to an American base nearby, and stood guard while they washed off the grime of days traveled without bathing. Then they returned to the "autobahn," where they hitchhiked again!

This "autobahn" had a lot of traffic, consisting mainly of American jeeps, because a football game was being played in a city situated on the road to Berlin. Finally a couple of officers stopped. They told Louise and Jacqueline that they were on their way to Berlin to attend a party being held two days later. After thoroughly examining their identity papers and their military orders, the officers decided to give them a ride, stopping in Giessen for the night before going on to Berlin.

It was still cold and drizzling, the back seat of the jeep was hard and offered little protection from the wind and the rain, and the noise prevented conversation. When they reached Giessen, all four climbed out of the jeep. One of the officers looked at Louise, and because she was short and female, asked her, "Are you really a doctor? If so, can you tell why my arm is so itchy?" Louise looked at his arm. The specific tunnel pattern made it obvious that he had scabies. The American officers were already not very friendly, but after that they were hardly civil!

The women were taken to a house to sleep and eat, and told they would be picked up at eight the next morning. The room had two beds and was in an unheated building saturated with a horrible smell of decay, had a cold shower and several clean towels. Later in the day they were directed to a mess hall, where they were glad to have a meal. The night was long and they did not feel safe. The next day the ride was very long, and they were very cold in the open jeep. Before they reached Berlin, cars were held up for a long time at a Russian checkpoint. Finally, after carefully looking at all the documents, some of which were upside down, the Russian police guards told the American officers and their passengers to go ahead. Snow started falling and it became dark very early. They finally reached a house in Berlin's American zone. Jacqueline and Louise asked if they could use the telephone to call their assigned hospital in North Berlin, which was in the French zone and ask to be picked up. The French at the hospital answered that no vehicle could cross the Russian zone at such an hour, and told them to call later. U.S. personnel crowded the house in the American zone where the jeep drivers had taken the women because there was a party for an officer returning to America. Most of the people were already drunk when Louise and Jacqueline arrived. After a while they begged to leave, being very tired, with red eyes and noses running from the long exposure to cold and wind in the rear seat of the jeep. One officer generously offered his room. The sheets on the large bed they shared were not clean, but there were toilets and a shower. There was no hot water, as usual. Since they had traveled a number of days without much washing or changing underwear and outerwear, they felt very filthy and enjoyed the facilities anyway!

In the morning, Jacqueline and Louise could smell bacon and were invited to a lush American breakfast. The officers who gave them a ride and a room were not there, but others kindly found them a telephone where they could speak again to someone at the French hospital. The hospital personnel could not get anyone to come and get them because traveling to and returning from the American zone required crossing the Russian zone twice, and they had very little gasoline to spare for cars. The small amount available was needed for ambulances. One American officer volunteered to do the paperwork that would enable an American driver to use a jeep to get them across Berlin through the Russian zone, and into the French zone to reach the French hospital.

While they crossed Berlin they had their first look at the devastation of what was once a beautiful city. Buildings were in shambles everywhere, streets were full of debris and the river carried debris and corpses. A church tower looked as if it had

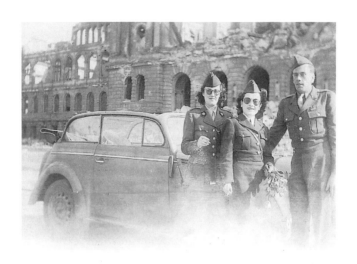

**Jacqueline and Louise in Berlin, winter 1945–46:
ruins of the city.**

been melted down. It was very frightening and sad. People were walking around aimlessly; women dressed in rags were picking up debris and stones. Finally they arrived at the French Military Hospital of Greater Berlin, and were welcomed by the chief physician, Colonel Lepine. It was November 11, 1945, the anniversary of the armistice of the First World War. The hospital, located in the French zone of Berlin in Reinickendorf Teichstrasse 65, was also called Louis Pasteur Hospital of Berlin. There was no pharmacist; the previous one had left the week before Jacqueline's arrival. She checked the very small inventory of pharmaceutical products and was given the key to the cupboard where the narcotics were kept, which she also checked. In November, 1945, there were no antibiotics, only sulfamides, and most widely used modern medications had yet to be developed.

The newly arrived physician, Louise, and pharmacist, Jacqueline, were shown the temporary room they had to share.

The room was located above the surgical block and had a bathroom with a shower and toilet. After taking showers, which burned, not from heat but from the horrendous concentration of chlorine, they emerged clean but red as lobsters and itchy. They enjoyed changing to clean uniforms because, thanks to Colonel Lechaux, their cantine had reached the hospital ahead of them. Their next experience was to eat dinner at the mess hall. There was nothing resembling a welcome! Most of the men sneered at them, except the Catholic chaplain who later became their savior when they refused to go to the mess hall, as the food was nauseating, the alcohol plentiful, and the atmosphere chilling!

The following day Jacqueline met her German laboratory technicians and listened to many promises that the hospital would get a clinical laboratory. Louise and Jacqueline both went to the patients' wards. They were not welcome there either. The hospital was old, had many separate buildings and was surrounded by a high stone wall. Patients were hospitalized in large wards, with beds on both sides, and no privacy! Several courtyards had to be crossed to go from one building to another. The bombings had damaged many roofs and many walls, and when the weather was windy, one had to watch for flying debris when crossing these yards.

A few days after their arrival they were visited by a couple of U.S. Air Force pilots who had heard of these two "frenchies" at the hospital. The pilots took Jacqueline and Louise to have dinner at Tempelhof, the Berlin airport in the American zone. They ate in groups of ten; the food was delectable. They were given some crackers and army rations, so the following evening they had a picnic in their room.

Life was very monotonous and unproductive; there were still no laboratory facilities or medications available. The narcotics had vanished overnight from the locked cupboard. There was little progress with the patients, who, for the most part, were pathetic displaced people who could not speak French, English, Spanish or German. Most of these patients had chronic malnutrition and tuberculosis. Among the outpatients that were French troops, there were many who had scabies and either gonorrhea or worse—syphilis—and there was no cure then!

Finally, by mid-December, Jacqueline had a small clinical laboratory. The weather was warmer. While in Paris on a furlough, Louise had met a very charming, very young American Air Force officer, Bob, who was a pilot with his quarters at the Tempelhof airport. Bob gave her numerous invitations to the military mess hall. After many months cooped up in their Berlin hospital, Louise and Jacqueline finally decided to inspect the heart of the black market at the Tiergarten. At that black market heaven, the exchanges were entirely made with cigarettes. German currency was not accepted because it was heavily devalued. They came back with a few items, which they kept for many years. Some weeks later Louise and Jacqueline were invited to a British club for dinner, but unhappily the food there was very tasteless.

Every now and then, Jacqueline received letters from Simone, who was in the U.S.A., and also from friends in Paris. Her parents and grandmother had returned to Neris-Les Bains, where they were better off than in Paris, having more food and also some heat. December 12 and 13 were Louise and Jacqueline's birthdays—but the depressing environment made celebration difficult.

Finally the Berlin medical community, including the French, the American, the British, the Russians, and even the Germans, got somewhat organized—and frequently Louise and Jacqueline could go to various hospitals and universities to listen to lectures and see presentation of patients with interesting medical problems. They were also able to eat outside of the hospital! The remaining medical personnel that the hospital chief promised, a pharmacist and a physician, never showed up.

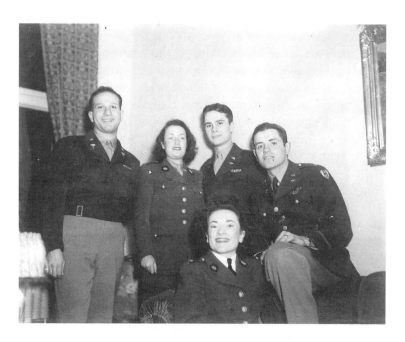

Tempelhof, in Berlin. From left to right: a pilot, Jacqueline, a pilot, Bob and his fiancée, Louise (in front), 1945.

The food was not any better, and Jacqueline wrote home to ask for packages of food and books. Louise's boyfriend, Bob, often flew to Paris and could pick up the packages. Luckily the two hospital chaplains (curés) were kind; they even had champagne for both Louise and Jacqueline's birthdays.

The year was over. No new pharmacists were coming, the laboratory technicians were leaving, and the new head physician was in the army, and was ferocious. His name was Colonel Béjard.

Louise and Jacqueline had a luxurious Christmas meal at Tempelhof airport. After a U.S. military jeep took them back to their quarters, there was a commotion in their hospital. Three American officers had been told that the French medics had a party. As the Americans had been dropped off and had no car, the French were responsible for getting them safely through the Russian zone and back to the American zone. With great difficulty, Jacqueline got them an ambulance for the promise of a full tank of gasoline after they got in the U.S. zone. They got very little sleep that night and were heavily criticized by Colonel Béjard—as if they had invited the three American officers! And so Jacqueline's year began with minimal responsibilities, mostly paperwork and dispensing of pharmaceuticals. Nothing changed for Louise professionally—except, perhaps, she had more patients to take care of.

On New Year's Eve, Louise was with Bob and Jacqueline in Tempelhof, but Jacqueline had the blues, with thoughts of Tuoc—and somehow she found herself in tears. An officer sitting at their table took her away to be kind and talk with her. His name was Captain Ritz and he was much older than Jacqueline. She never forgot him and his concern. In January, Louise and Jacqueline received some packages from France, with a little food, which was scarce all over Europe! Many packages arrived empty. In addition, personal items like perfume, soap, etc., were stolen from the women's room. Work was not rewarding. Jacqueline was sent all over the city to collect water samples to analyze. The jeeps were open and it was bitter cold. Between working hours they managed to save some cigarettes to return to the Tiergarten and do some bartering, or they took the train or the subway to go to various military compounds to see some movies—mostly to get out!

Jacqueline was asked to give lectures to the nursing personnel concerning disinfection, without any books on the premises to help substantiate what she had memorized! She also had more help from German laboratory technicians who did not speak French or English, but had laboratory skills. Jacqueline needed to have some bacterial culture media (Loeffler media) for her laboratory. She was given a pass to go to a slaughter-house in the Russian zone, to obtain sterile blood from cattle in order to have fresh, sterile blood plasma. She took many bottles with screw tops, dutifully sterilized. When she got to the Russian plant they had to walk through rivers of blood; none of the Russian workers knew how to open a screw-top bottle. By the time she returned and processed the blood she had obtained, all of it was contaminated, and she could not prepare the needed bacterial culture media. She was also sent to what was left of the Schering Laboratories to get medication for the increasing number of military personnel who had scabies. Incredibly, there were many people still working in the pharmaceutical plant, which was partially destroyed by the bombings.

There was some fun. Bob, the U.S. pilot who wanted to marry Louise, continued to invite them to Tempelhof for meals, parties, and dances. The girls tasted their first hamburger—so big and so good! There was even a dance in their hospital, with very little food but lots of unspecified alcohol—*la gnole*—to drink. Even the Russian officers came. It was hot, and the men were permitted to take off their jackets, but the Russians could not because they were wearing nothing underneath! Louise and Jacqueline were waiting to get out of the military service, and in mid-February, 1945, were told that all AFATS were demobilized except those in the Medical Corps! No luck! But life was getting somewhat better. There were movies; they were invited to listen to *Madame Butterfly* at the German opera house. The theater was beautiful and the show magnificent, even among the ruins. Berlin was getting cleaned up from debris, and public transportation was slowly becoming available.

Around the end of February, Jacqueline's brother-in-law, Jean, had suggested that her future might be better if she emigrated to the U.S.A. and so she made a decision to leave for America eight to ten months later. She was very sure that with her diplomas and numerous laboratory skills she could easily find work. As her family had moved back to Paris to a small apartment, with no space for her, she did not feel guilty about leaving them. The thought of such a new beginning in her future helped her in the daily routine. In addition, Jacqueline's sister, Simone, was expecting again! Jacqueline received a letter from Tuoc. He told her he was leaving for Vietnam. She wrote back to encourage him to go and fulfill his dreams—but it was very hard for her to accept.

Louise and Jacqueline had few chances to spent money; instead they sent their military salaries to their parents, who needed their help because resettling in France was financially very difficult. When March arrived, life became more and more militarized. There were no guests or passes, and things became very difficult for Louise and Bob, who were planning their wedding. So Jacqueline made an official request to get an apartment away from the hospital, where there was a full collaboration between male personnel and German women, who climbed the high wall surrounding the hospital and were often found in the patients' beds! By the end of March they had an apartment very close to the hospital. The apartment was one where the previous German hospital chief had lived before but was kicked out because he was a Nazi, and neither Louise nor Jacqueline had any guilty feelings about taking it over. The apartment was heated, and even had hot water, and there was enough coal for a little while. They cooked their lunches, had a telephone installed, and hired a cleaning lady! They really enjoyed the comfort and privacy, but their lives were very boring. It was snowing again, and they had very little work to do. They asked their families to send some novels and some tea! Time moved slowly, but finally April came. The weather improved and they were able to venture out further into the city, on the public transportation that was available.

Louise and Jacqueline were officially demobilized in June, but because they were not replaced they had to stay in their jobs. The quality of their life steadily improved; they had more food and more outings. June and July went by; they began getting ready to leave. One fond but absurd memory was when the American Medical group gave the hospital some supplies of penicillin. Jacqueline was elated to have the drug to treat her patients! But then Colonel Béjard and a Russian physician came to the pharmacy, and the colonel requested the stock of penicillin and gave it to the Russians, although not necessarily willingly. How the Russians learned about the American gift is a mystery.

When September came, Louise and Jacqueline finally returned to Paris by train—very slowly! So, Jacqueline and Louise had finally returned from Berlin. Tuoc was waiting, and Suzanne was very insistent that Jacqueline say yes to Tuoc's proposal of marriage . . . and for Jacqueline, the decision to leave had been very, very difficult. The years spent with Tuoc were still wonderful memories—they were the happiest years of her life.

VII

Returning to Paris after the Nazi Occupation

After their demobilization and return to the apartment on rue du Theatre in Paris, Louise and Jacqueline settled as well as the disorganized economy permitted. The city was still in disarray. There were still food and fuel shortages, and public services and transportation were still disorganized. There was not much improvement in the comfort of life! In addition, people had no money because a new currency was replacing the old franc. During the winter of 1946–47, Jacqueline concentrated on studying to get through the examinations necessary for obtaining her pharmacist license. She also needed to obtain a certification of her four-year hospital intership, describing her clinical laboratory skills and her pharmaceutical-manufacturing abilities. She had been delayed in taking these tests because as long as the German occupation lasted she could not register because she was Jewish. The winter was harsh and her apartment still had no central heat. At the same time, Louise finished her M.D. thesis, describing how the newly isolated Vitamin D was toxic when given to newborn babies in quantities that were too large. She started working for a pharmaceutical company, Roussel UCLA, while finishing her thesis.

Life in Paris was drab and uncomfortable. Jacqueline studied in her cold living room, heated by the same small coal furnace she had used during the war and Nazi occupation. She

61

even got burns on her back because she sat so close to the heater! Friends and relatives had not yet returned to Paris, and many had disappeared. Money was in short supply; the appearance of the new franc made it hard for black-marketers to enjoy their profits. Thankfully, Jacqueline had the friendship of her neighbors, Henriette Lechaux and her daughters, to cheer her up. Her daughter Renée married a professional military man whom she met at a party for military personnel, which included her father. For the wedding she wore a white net dress that had been made for Jacqueline for a fancy dance party before the war.

Everyone was very thin. Suzanne and Gaston were trying to cope with their losses and start new lives. When Jacqueline talked about going to America, they were dismayed with the idea of having both daughters away, but thought that it might be better for their future. Even in 1947, very little progress had been made improving the look and atmosphere of Paris; the city was filthy and its upkeep neglected. Many industrial plants had exploded after being set on fire by the French when the Germans arrived in Paris, and also when Paris was liberated. This occurred mostly at La Halle au Vin (the wine hall), resulting in clouds of soot that made every building in the city look drab, miserable, dark, sad and dirty.

At this time, Simone was settled in the USA. She had had several miscarriages but was expecting again. Her husband Jean suggested that it would be a good idea for Jacqueline to come to the USA after getting her pharmacy license. She could help Simone with the new baby and could find interesting employment. Jacqueline made all the necessary arrangements to emigrate. She obtained letters from Jean's family showing that they would help financially, if needed. She went to the U.S. consulate for an interview to obtain approval and get an immigration visa, with the help of her pharmacy background. In May of 1947, she took her first plane to the USA. After a few days with Jean's family in New York City, she took a bus to Schoharie, a tiny village near Schenectady, in New York state. Simone and Jean were both working in Schenectady for the General Electric Company. They could not find lodging there so they rented a small apartment in Schoharie, over a bus stop. After she arrived, Jacqueline tried to help her sister to remain mostly in bed until the baby was born, which occurred on June 23, 1947. The weather was lovely, flowers were blooming everywhere, and Jacqueline was enchanted by the countryside and by her niece Annie! Even so, she kept thinking about Tuoc . . . how he would have enjoyed coming with her. She tried to forget her loneliness and to look ahead.

VIII

America

Part I: Before Texas

Jacqueline was pleased that it was probably because of her help the baby was fat and healthy. Sadly there was not enough money for her to stay with Simone, Jean and Annie. The family hardly had enough money to survive. Jacqueline was still very emotionally torn. She still loved Tuoc but did not want to destroy his dreams, afraid that later he would be very unhappy!

Through her brother-in-law, she met many handsome, young engineers working for the General Electric Company. She had many dates but felt much more mature and educated than most of the men, and thought no relationships with any of them could exist. There was one exception: Seymour, a man who, during the war, had acquired life experience outside the USA and knowledge of European civilization. He was very handsome, tall and lean. She dated him for a long time and would have married him if he had asked, but he did not. He was afraid of her French and Jewish background! To this day Seymour remains a faithful friend, sending Jacqueline cards for Valentine's Day and other holidays. She realized later that he had made the right choice by marrying an old friend who gave him a secure, protected life and was totally devoted to him. In addition, she later learned from Simone that Seymour had a long list of girlfriends around the world!

While she was visiting her family in Schenectady, Jacqueline went to the laboratory of the local hospital to help, and to learn the American laboratory terminology. She volunteered at the hospital as a laboratory technician for several hours daily, and worked in a maternity hospital as well. Through a placement agency she found a job in a small hospital with two hundred and fifty beds, in Mineola, Long Island. She reached the place by bus, carrying only a small piece of luggage. When she arrived she had to work around the clock in the clinical laboratory. She lived in a room in the nurses' home. She started taking blood at seven in the morning and was on call most weekends and evenings. Her salary was so low that she could not even afford a small table radio.

When she took the job she intended to work nights in the laboratory and go to a fashion design school in New York City during the day. Instead, she worked nights and days in a very dishonest laboratory, having to sign for results of clinical tests that were not performed! She resigned as soon as her fees to the placement agency were paid and she found another job. Not only was the job disheartening, the hospital and the living facilities were poor. Mineola was, and still is, a very unappealing suburb, and since she had no car there she had no resources for relaxation. She left as soon as she was hired as the chief of the clinical laboratory in a hospital which specialized in thyroid pathology, in Sayre, Pennsylvania. The village of Sayre was very small and she had to live at the hospital, across from the morgue, in a huge room with a big bathtub in the middle! She started at a laboratory, at six-thirty in the morning, going to various patients' rooms to draw blood samples. All the personnel were friendly and helpful, and the techniques were good. She got off at three o'clock in the afternoon, and then she either walked to the high school to find tennis partners or climbed up the hills above the Susquehanna River for long walks. The landscape was beautiful. Every other weekend the laboratory personnel drew blood from high school youngsters for the local blood bank. The Sayre Hospital was very progressive, because at that time blood banks were new!

The other weekends, when she was not on-call, she took the bus to Schenectady, where Simone, Jean and Annie had moved into a very small frame house, lent to them by a friend of Simone's. The winter was cold, and the hills and forest were covered with snow. One night in Schenectady when she was left alone with the baby, the coal in the cellar stove stopped burning. The house was rapidly getting cold and she panicked, as Ann was no more than six months old. It was two in the morning when she called one of her General Electric boyfriends for help. He came immediately and fixed the problem very efficiently! During the winter months, Jacqueline was trying to find a way to go back to school to acquire an American education, as she was determined to do clinical research, primarily in pharmacology.

Jean's aunt and uncle lived in New York City. They were wonderful, erudite people, and they helped Jacqueline sort out her future, but since they had not been educated in the U.S., their help regarding the academic structure of the country was limited. Having no advice from university people, she refused an offer to attend graduate school at Yale, not realizing the school's prestige, and instead accepted two-year credit toward a pharmacy degree at Union College in Albany, New York.

Jacqueline still has a lovely memory of a visit with a patient she had in Sayre. Knowing she did not have a family nearby, the patient asked her to spend the weekend with her at her home. There was a clambake on the beach, and the food was cooked the American Indian way, on a stack of wood: layers of corn, oysters and lobsters! The following day, despite her protests that she had never learned to ride a horse, her hostess put Jacqueline on the back of a large, aging mare, who took her all around the village, where apples were picked to make cider, and the air was saturated by the smell. The rest of the day was a blur due to a lot of drinking at the local club.

Jacqueline's parents were finally financially able to travel from Paris to visit their daughters and meet their granddaughter and grandson. After visiting with Simone, who was recovering from the birth of a baby boy, Alain, by Caesarian section, they decided to come see where their younger daughter was working—but Sayre had no hotel in 1947, so they were invited by a local Protestant minister to spend a night in his home. They were very surprised and embarrassed, being of another faith. And the bed was so high they needed a stool to get on it!

When fall came, Jacqueline had to find lodging in Albany, to start college. She found an adequate room in a private home, about half a mile from the school. For breakfast she was entitled to two cups of coffee and two slices of buttered toast—but no more! She had to find work to pay for her room, food, books and tuition. Saint Peter's Hospital, in Albany, managed by The Sisters of the Poor, needed a clinical laboratory technician from three o'clock in the afternoon until any time needed to perform all the tests required at the clinical laboratory, and also for cross-matching blood for transfusions. At that time there were very few blood banks. The job had a bonus: an evening meal at the cafeteria.

Albany was an appealing town, situated in the beautiful New York countryside, but without money or a car, Jacqueline could not enjoy it, nor could she enjoy the bucolic scenery of New York State. In addition, she had very little time between completing her course load and the chores in the hospital. She had to wait for busses in the cold and wet winters, when snow kept falling, and even with boots she was always cold! But it was so much better than Paris in 1940; in Albany houses were warm, there was plenty of warm clothing and plenty of food, and there was no threat of being arrested!

Jacqueline had so little free time that between the school, her job, her sister and her sister's babies, she went on very few dates. In addition, her pharmacy schoolmates were too young to date, and the men she had previously dated were too far away! She briefly dated a law student, Bob, who wanted to become a reporter. He took Jacqueline to one of the Finger Lakes to visit his family, but she felt like such a fraud among his family, who were farmers, that she stopped dating him. After this she had an affair with a medical student, Sherman. Neither Jacqueline nor Sherman had any intention of a serious relationship. Unfortunately, Jacqueline became pregnant; Sherman's family was frantic and arranged a back-street abortion. That was the end of her romances with students! The good sisters of Saint Peter's Hospital wanted her to attend little parties so she could meet a nice gentleman. Again, she would have felt out of place. She took lonely walks when the weather was good. One afternoon, on a very foggy day, she was walking along a road when a car ran her off, and someone opened a door and tried to grab her! Never having time to read newspapers and their ghastly reports of rape and murder, she was not even scared.

In school, the courses went smoothly, and she got very good grades, except for her business course. To overcome this failure, the dean of the college gave Jacqueline private tutoring for a while on Saturday mornings—he was very kind! All the students of the pharmacy school were so young that it was difficult for her to make friends, but luckily she became friends with a young architect, Jules. She met Jules at the home of his aunt, who entertained students of pharmacy, medicine, law and architecture every week. All these schools were in the same vicinity. Jacqueline went with Jules to many antique stores in the countryside where she bought early American furniture that she still has. She enjoyed sight-seeing in New England's quaint villages and countryside. She went to see her family in Schenectady, and ate good meals at every opportunity. During her second year in Albany, she was able to move to a basement apartment in a brownstone, sharing the bath and garden with an attractive and friendly girl, Irene, who worked for the telephone company (AT&T). Finally, life was easier, until Jacqueline, unable to find a blood donor for a patient, gave her own blood in a volume too large for her weight. It took a terrible toll on her energy! Finally the two years were over and she had a formal graduation with cap and gown for the first time. Simone came, and it was very festive! Jacqueline took the New York Pharmacy Board examination a few weeks later and made the top of the list!

She returned for a while to live with Simone and to enjoy her little niece, and get to know Alain, who was born in February, earlier than expected. She tried to help her sister, which was easy because they also had the assistance of a very efficient elderly black woman. She had white hair and brown skin, which was amazing to Annie, who had never met anyone who was African-American. She was the first black person Jacqueline ever knew personally and loved.

Money was short and Jacqueline had to search for a paying job. She received an offer from Johns Hopkins Hospital in Baltimore. She visited and found that the city had rows of brick houses like the charming brownstones in New York City and the position offered was very appealing. But then she took a plane to Wilmington, North Carolina, for another interview. On a warm spring day, she was taken to a huge park full of magnolias, azaleas and other blooming plants of all colors and shapes—this was so wonderful after the drabness of Albany! It was love at first sight, so she signed up for the job of head pharmacist in a small, independent hospital, where she would do the buying of all the hospital medications, and the dispensing of the prescriptions given to the patients. She did not have a clinical laboratory to take care of anymore! She rented a small apartment across the street from the hospital. She learned to drive, but never to get drunk at the country club, which was the greatest attraction in the small town. She promptly took the examination for the North Carolina State Board of Pharmacy. The beach was ten miles from her apartment. By starting out for work at seven in the morning, she could go daily, year-round, to the wonderful Wrightsville Beach, around three in the afternoon, where she could swim and walk, or take the car around the beautiful coastline to Cape Fear and other historical sites.

Jacqueline soon learned that in the south, black people were treated strangely. They had their own part of town and their own drinking fountain. It was appalling!

She made some nice friends, and was thrown into the arms of the local pharmacist, Lawrence Britt. Unfortunately he was gay, and died of cancer very soon after she left Wilmington. But he was very kind, and Jacqueline befriended his family, who lived a short distance away in a very small town. The countryside was lovely. It had huge trees with Spanish moss, grand mansions from the past, and little towns where everyone knew each other! Many weekends she went with Lawrence to his sister's house. His sister, known as Miss Edna, was married to a lawyer. They would pick up his other sister, Gwen, who was married to a physician, and then all would go to a Baptist Church service. Following the service, dinner was served behind the church by Miss Suzie, a black woman, with the help of another older black woman, Miss Eva. These little towns had no restaurants or fast food, but there were wonderful pork barbeques in the black section of town.

After a year and a half at work, she met a pharmaceutical company representative, Charles, who courted her. But he was very boring, and also ten years younger than she. One of the hospital board members had a young daughter, Eleanor, who learned that the pharmacist was a French woman, so she invited Jacqueline to the Junior League, to high school festivities, and more. Jacqueline was told by the hospital director to accept the invitations! She found herself dancing the French cancan at the high school, and attending other social gatherings that she hated. She thought that Eleanor and Charles might be happy to meet. Eventually they got married and the pressure of a constant social life became unbearable for Jacqueline! It was time to quit the small southern paradise. At about the same time, she met another drug manufacturer's representative, Steve, who was about her age, good looking, and had all the charm of a southern gentleman. Jacqueline fell for him, and for his false promises to marry her after he divorced a mentally-ill, estranged wife!

Jacqueline resigned from her job and went to Paris to visit her parents. She returned on the French ocean-liner, the *Ile de France*, where she got a taste of luxury. She even won a ping-pong tournament and still has the silver cup! She returned to Wilmington to pack and say farewell to her social friends. She was not in the U.S. for such frivolities. Social life in Paris with Tuoc would have been much better. She looked for another school or teaching hospital so she could work and return to school.

She read stories about the magnificent medical center that was taking shape in Houston, Texas. She had also read about the new University of Houston, so she sent off many applications and was accepted at both the University of Houston and M.D. Anderson Hospital. She left Wilmington, shipping her belongings to be stowed away, taking as much as possible in her green convertible, and making a date with Steve in New Orleans. She took small roads toward Louisiana and met Steve, spending a few romantic days in the old city before taking the old Route 90 toward Houston, not even having a map of that city and not knowing anyone there! She was in good mental shape after visiting her parents during the summer, and returning on the *Ile de France*, traveling first-class, courtesy of her father, as already mentioned above. Being broke and alone did not bother Jacqueline and she still vaguely believed that Steve was going to marry her!

Jacqueline obtained her citizenship five years after she arrived in the U.S. and then went to Paris to visit her family. By that time they were more comfortable financially. They took her all over Italy on one visit, and they also took her on a lengthy trip to Israel. Simone joined them for part of this trip. Another year, when Morocco was still a French colony, they had spent several weeks touring the marvelous country, traveling around in a chauffeured car! Most of Jacqueline's vacations were spent in Geneva, where Jean and Simone lived for many years in a small house near Lake Leman, in a village called Vandoeuvres. The whole family stayed together for two to four weeks, enjoying the children, Ann and Alain, the pleasures of boating, and the spectacular fireworks on the lake.

Part II: Texas

Jacqueline arrived in Houston on a sweltering weekday in September, 1953. She was totally ignorant of the topography of the city, and stopped in a motel on route 90, on the east side of the city. Houston was a small town then; it had no freeways. There were grid-patterned streets crossed by railroad tracks. The morning following her arrival, after a restful sleep, she found the University of Houston, which was also on the east side of town. The entrance was on a wide dirt road; the back faced another dirt road across from a slaughterhouse and packing plant which smelled very bad! She located the pharmacy school building. She hoped that she could find a room on the campus and also wanted to ask when the lectures started. After finally locating someone at the pharmacy building, she was told that there was no dormitory room available for her and to come back a week later for registration. There was a phone booth near the main entrance of the school, and luckily another student was also there looking for a place to live. He had located a small apartment complex within walking distance of the university. They went to inquire about it; and Jacqueline was immediately able to rent an apartment. The apartment was built like a town house, with two stories, a walled garden, a garage and two entrances. The kitchen opened into the parking area. There was also a large landscaped area. The rent was one hundred dollars a month. A week later she started studying at the University of Houston where the Pharmacology Department was very efficient and well staffed.

At the apartment complex there were two families with whom Jacqueline became friends. One was an engineer and his wife, Amelia. Jacqueline and Amelia did artwork together, mostly mosaics. The other was a family of four: the father, of whom she saw very little, the mother, Della, who had a sweet, friendly, sincere soul, and treated Jacqueline as if she were a part of her family, and two boys, Bob and Bill. Jacqueline became very attached to Bill, with whom she shared her artistic activities. Later on, when she met the man she would eventually marry, Bob, she had to give up the friendship with Bill because Bob was jealous!

Jacqueline was appalled by the schism between white and black people she found in Houston and found it was the same in Texas as in North Carolina. In addition, white people and black people in Texas also hated the Mexicans! What about being the "United States?" Jacqueline wondered. Jacqueline's only experience of racial hatred was the Nazis' hatred of the Jews. She was ignorant of racism's history and politics.

At the University of Houston, the pharmacology program was outstanding and demanding. She kept busy doing numerous and lengthy laboratory experiments to assess the effect of drugs on various animal species; these experiments often took all night. In addition, in order to survive financially she taught physiology and biochemistry to future optometrists and, at what was then the Methodist Hospital, future nurses. The Methodist hospital at that time was downtown, an easy ride from Jacqueline's apartment. Jacqueline also worked in various pharmacies for a dollar an hour, after getting her Texas State Board Pharmacy license. Socially, the school had little to offer, but some of the pharmacy faculty tried to match Jacqueline up with one of the teachers, who was an alcoholic. The Alliance Francaise allowed her to meet very friendly French engineers from Schlumberger Company, primarily because her father was at the Ecole Polytechnique at the same time as Conrad Schlumberger, so his name was known by some of the older people working in Houston. This gave her a chance to make some new friends.

But Jacqueline had little time or money for a social life. She wanted to swim, play tennis, and study. She was lucky to know a member of the Cork Club, who gave her a pass to the Shamrock Hotel, which had a beautiful swimming pool. By then she had completely forgotten Steve and his tales. There were numerous tennis courts at the university but they were always closed. She could not find tennis partners, and a French girl she had met at the university suggested she could call one of her male acquaintances, who might want to play. Jacqueline met this fellow and it was love at first sight. His name was Bob Walker.

Instead of playing tennis they went to lunch in a seafood restaurant on South Main Street, that had been transformed from a boat. Then they swam at Bob's apartment. The following weekend he invited her to go with him to Corpus Christi, where he had work to do. They stayed in a now defunct hotel on the beach and then stayed together for twenty years, until his untimely death! Bob was tall, with wide shoulders, built like a stevedore, with no neck! He had a wonderful personality and a fantastic memory, and he loved to talk. He was just starting to get heavy. Jacqueline was terribly thin, and because of that, even with her tennis games and plenty of swimming on weekends, she had back and neck pain. She tried to exercise more to compensate for muscle weakness. Finally she put on a few pounds and felt much better.

Bob showed her the beauty of the Gulf of Mexico, and of Galveston. They rented small boats all around the island, and Jacqueline learned to fish and to catch blue crabs. She was hooked forever! Houston had very few restaurants, and no fast food facilities. Texas did not allow the sale of alcoholic beverages in public places, only in private clubs! Some of these clubs were elegant and had good food, but were all financially unavailable for Jacqueline and Bob, and Jacqueline hated their restrictions: no blacks and no Jews unless they were very rich, such as the owners of the Neiman Marcus stores. So Jacqueline usually cooked at her apartment. The food choices were meager. Butter was always salted, the bread white and mushy. French cheeses were unknown here, as well as many other French delicacies.

Two years later Jacqueline graduated from the University of Houston Pharmacology Department. Her thesis described the location of brain receptors for the first of a new generation of brain-modifying drugs, chlorpromazine. She worked on rodents, cats, dogs and monkeys, but Jacqueline was not satisfied. Only clinical research on humans could fulfill her dreams, so she would eventually return to graduate school. But she could not do so until she could afford to pay for school again. She had to earn some money.

Jacqueline took a job as a clinical laboratory supervisor at M.D. Anderson Hospital. While she was there she did chemistry research on thyroid pathology and analyzed many samples of blood and urine from patients that had been treated with radioactive iodine. She audited an excellent course on radioactivity; it was held at M.D. Anderson and was taught by a physicist. To carry out more research on endocrinology, she induced a fibrosarcoma in a colony of white rats. She was very interested in examining possible changes in the endocrine system of rats bearing the tumors. The tumors were brought on with multiple methycholanthrene applications on the necks of young rats, in addition to radiation exposure; they were transferred to new colonies of rats every three months. After several transfers it became more malignant and the rats died within twenty to twenty-two days.

After more than a year at M.D. Anderson, Jacqueline had an opportunity to visit a laboratory at the College de France that was well-known for its work on the synthesis of radioactive thyroid hormones, under the direction of Professor Roche and his wife. She went so she could learn about techniques related to measurements and synthesis of these hormones, and the use of radioactive iodine. The short life span of the rats bearing tumors made it difficult to leave her laboratory for any length of time until she found an assistant. Then she was able to go to Paris, where she stayed with her parents.

Early in the morning she took the bus to go to the Latin Quarter at the College de France where she worked every day for a month, happy to acquire new knowledge to bring back to her Houston hospital laboratory. In Professor Roche's laboratory, she was appalled by the very careless use of highly radioactive iodine, and had a quarrel with Roche, who was very uncooperative and rude. Eventually his wife apologized for him. On the first day after she returned to M.D. Anderson Hospital, she was called to Personnel where she was informed that she had used her vacation-time for three years! Utterly disgusted, she resigned immediately. Later she was asked by the head of the hospital to establish a pharmacology research laboratory. She spent a few days drawing up a list of the necessary facilities. The extent of the work to set up a valid drug-screening laboratory was far above what that physician expected, and the whole idea was forgotten. At the hospital, Jacqueline met Dr. Ilse

Mannheimer, who specialized in the care of women with terminal cancer. They remained friends until Ilse's death.

A Baylor College of Medicine endocrinologist, Dr. Marc Moldawer, was interested in Jacqueline's research and hired her to work in his laboratory.

During the time she worked for Dr. Moldawer, her relationship with Bob Walker had problems. She became pregnant, and once again the would-be father had no desire to have a child. This time it was because Bob had a daughter from his previous marriage and could not even pay for her support, therefore it was out of the question to have a baby. He threatened to commit suicide if she didn't end the pregnancy, so she did. The abortion was done poorly and Jacqueline had to be hospitalized for a D and C at Methodist Hospital. Jacqueline recovered quickly and was able to return to work after a couple of days. Dr. Moldawer became aware of Jacqueline's desire to get a degree that would allow her to do clinical research of her own, and very kindly helped her to enroll as a graduate student at Baylor College of Medicine. The school was small, containing only about twenty male medical students, and for the first time in the school's history, there were three women enrolled in graduate studies. Most of the teaching was good except some lectures that were somewhat outdated and too theoretical. Jacqueline's first adviser wanted her to work on his research project, but she refused. She was having difficulty in Houston until she was invited to visit the staff at the Pharmacology Department at the Texas Medical School of Galveston, the oldest in Texas. She nearly bought a house there, but then a fellow Frenchman and researcher, Dr. Roger Guillemin, offered to be the advisor for her graduate work, and to sponsor her research at Baylor. So she stayed in Houston.

When she started graduate school she found a lump in one of her breasts. Seemingly overnight, she had to have a lumpectomy. Though it was benign, it was a psychological shock! It happened during the summer, the students had no health insurance! This frightening state of affairs was promptly amended by one of the school physicians, Dr. Harry Lipscomb. After several years of graduate school and some teaching, she finally got her degree. Her thesis described the endocrinological damage produced by a fibrosarcoma in rats. Now she needed money, and she had to look for a job!

In 1964 she was hired at The Institute for Rehabilitation and Research (TIRR), which had been a center for the care of poliomyelitis patients, then became one of the rehabilitation centers set up by the U.S. government to care for patients paralyzed by spinal cord injuries. Bob and Jacqueline decided they could afford to get married, since Jacqueline had a small salary. The event was modest. They could not find a Justice of the Peace in Houston, so they rode toward Galveston, and stopped in Dickinson, where they were married. They spent the night at the now defunct Hotel Jack Tar!

Bob and Jacqueline bought a house on a street where Jacqueline's friend from M.D. Anderson, Dr. Ilse Mannheimer, had lived for ten years. It was wonderful. Within a year they had a swimming pool in the backyard and shortly afterwards they added a bedroom with a bath, where Jacqueline was hoping that her mother, now a widow, could live around the year. But Suzanne only came for visits; she didn't want to leave Paris.

The work at TIRR was fascinating. There was so much knowledge to acquire in physiology, pharmacology and endocrine function because patients with injuries at the cervical level, with a total transection of the spinal cord, were the perfect models to study as described by Claude Bernard in "The Isolated Encephalus."

Bob bought a small motor for the boats they rented in Galveston to go crabbing and fishing. After a while they had saved enough money to buy a small used boat, and then a bigger one. Jacqueline loved fishing but became seasick easily and did not like the idea of a larger boat with sleeping facilities. They were happy, but Bob drank too much, continuing a bad habit acquired during prohibition and his military life during the war in Europe. As Bob was getting fatter, Jacqueline became thinner. Houston was still a small town without freeways, and very few restaurants. There was a good Fine Arts Museum, and Jones Hall was built downtown for the symphony and ballet. The Medical Center was still easily accessible, and parking was free. The Rodeo was a big event; it was small and wonderful. Life was finally kind to Jacqueline.

At the TIRR, in 1965, Jacqueline requested the help of Dr. Nino Differanti, a specialist in collagen studies. He wanted to introduce Jacqueline to his wife, Marie Therese (MT), a Canadian, because he thought they could be friends. When Jacqueline met MT and her four children, they did become very close friends! Nino and Bob got along as well; which was a bonus. Later on, Charlotte, MT's mother, joined the household, and also became her friend. MT often came to dinner with her mother when Suzanne was visiting. To this day, MT is Jacqueline's closest, most erudite friend. She keeps abreast of what is going on in the world by being an avid reader of the *New York Times*. She is much younger than Jacqueline and became a real godsend much later in life by taking Jacqueline to the medical center for her medical problems. She is Jacqueline's guest nearly every Sunday evening. She understands French and is like a younger sister for Jacqueline, always giving sound advice. MT has an advanced degree in health care, so they have a great deal in common and can discuss medical problems, drug effects, etc. MT worked in public health and was able to bring many wonderful black women into the system.

Jacqueline often visited her family and her sister's family in Paris and Geneva. She was finally able to have elegant clothing, even though she often covered it up with white lab coats.

Most of the time she and Bob entertained their friends at home, as both loved to cook. By then they had acquired simple but nice furnishings, improving their old rustic house every year. Bob created a lovely landscape for the backyard, and for the garden plot that was visible from the living room. Jacqueline's parents visited them once a year. Bob adored Suzanne and Gaston.

On one trip to Paris, Jacqueline visited a distant cousin, Georges Klein. He was an artist, and had met many impressionists in his youth. He lived in a crumbling three-hundred-year-old house near the Sacred Heart Church, with a woman from Madagascar who was a model at one time. They told Jacqueline that her mother had rescued her brother-in-law, Georges Claus, from the prison of Drancy! Jacqueline had never heard anything about this, but her mother refused to tell her anything more, so how and when it was accomplished always remained a mystery.

Jacqueline's father died at age ninety-two. Her mother lived to be ninety-seven and visited Houston regularly until she was ninety-five. In addition to Bob's company, she also enjoyed the dog Toto, named after her father. Life went on after her parents' deaths. Jacqueline traveled often for her work, attending many conferences, but Bob always refused to go along. He did not like to spend money that he had not personally earned, and also didn't like not being the star of the show! Bob worked for several companies over the years, but could not get anything permanent; because of his previous illness he could never get health insurance! Jacqueline and Bob finally went to France together in 1975. Gaston was dead by then, but Suzanne enjoyed the visit and a glorious trip to southern France where they met Rosa in Cannes and Renée in Nice. Life was great!

To her great surprise, beginning in 1957, Jacqueline received a couple of letters from Tuoc. She did not want Bob to know about this because he would be upset and would not understand. Once, while visiting Suzanne in Paris, she met Tuoc at an art show. Even then he was accompanied by two body-guards! He wanted to visit Suzanne, but the bodyguards had to follow! Later, while she was still in Paris, Jacqueline met him again. He had arranged the meeting with Rosa and Marc to have dinner at their house in Choisy le Roi, near Paris. Throughout the evening, Tuoc constantly looked at his watch because he had to return to his communist quarters at a prearranged hour. In 1937, as an M.D. in Paris, he always looked very dandy. But at these meetings he wore miserable clothes and well-worn shoes with drooping white socks. Jacqueline kept all the letters from 1957 and the letters he subsequently wrote twenty years later from Vietnam and its communist satellites, until his death.

While Jacqueline was visiting her mother and sister in 1976, Dr. Mannheimer called to say that Bob was in the hospital and the diagnosis was not good. She made an emergency return to Houston. He died within two months, of pancreatic cancer. He was only sixty-two! That was the end of Jacqueline's happiness and fulfillment. Suzanne was still visiting in Houston and also missed him very much after he died.

One day, Jacqueline's ex-boyfriend from Schenectady, Seymour, whom she had met during her early years in America knocked on her door in Houston. Suzanne was visiting at the time and he took both of them to dinner. It was the beginning of a lasting relationship.

At TIRR, Jacqueline had a dreary, windowless office on the third floor of an adjoining building. It was a small improvement from originally being located in the basement of TIRR, in a room like a closet. She had a wonderful secretary who helped her to put research projects into writing and to write medical articles. Her office was near Dr. David Cardus's office. His wife, Paquita, who was a pharmacist, worked for him in the laboratory. Dr. Cardus had a young and pretty secretary named Elisabeth.

One day Elisabeth came to Jacqueline's office to ask questions about Paris, where she was planning to go to school to study French, while her husband, a plastic surgeon, had to stay in the intensive care unit of the Methodist Hospital around the clock, for his residency training program. Jacqueline gave her Suzanne's and Simone's addresses. Jacqueline's entire Parisian family fell in love with Elisabeth. She studied for four months at the Sorbonne. When Elisabeth returned to Houston, she thought she would go back to Mexico, when suddenly she learned that her marriage was over! So she divorced and lived alone in an apartment in Houston while recovering emotionally. After a while, Jacqueline asked Elisabeth to share her house; Elisabeth gave Jacqueline great moral and emotional support. Elisabeth dated, went to shows, took bicycle rides, and for a long time enjoyed the freedom of being single. Her company made Jacqueline's life far more pleasant.

One day Elisabeth met Jean Francois at a dinner arranged by mutual friends. Somehow a spark was lit in her heart and they started to date steadily. Jacqueline thought she was interfering with the romance because she was so often present when they courted, so she suggested that Elisabeth leave her house and rent an apartment by herself so the relationship could bloom—and it did. They were married. Seymour was at the ceremony. Jean Francois, a Belgian, had a cultural background similar to the French, and right away he became very good friends with Jacqueline. Later in life, the young couple bought a house near Jacqueline's and they are wonderful to her to this day. Jean Francois is extremely erudite, and teaches computer science at the University of Houston, where he is a fully tenured professor. Because he is from Belgium and Elisabeth's French is perfect, they all speak French when they are together. Jacqueline enjoys their company, and their proximity gives her a feeling of security, as both Ann and Alain are so far away as was Simone.

Finally, Jacqueline could afford the expense and the time to purchase nice clothing and an elegant car and travel throughout the world. After Bob's death, she was able to resume an old friendship with Bill McKenzie, who was her neighbor when she first arrived in Houston. Throughout all her years as a widow, Bill escorted her to activities related to fine art, and was always there to take care of her animals: Toto the dog, and Gigi the cat. But Bill is now getting old too! They share all artistic activities. Jacqueline's home is made cheerful by a wonderful fountain Bill constructed, which she admires from her living room, as well as a unique metal light fixture he crafted, which hangs in her entry hall.

At work, Jacqueline had a very efficient Cuban-American laboratory technician, Gladys. Little by little, Gladys acquired all the knowledge necessary to run Jacqueline's laboratory. She helped in the writing of research publications and came along to medical meetings. Eventually, Gladys was doing her own research, obtained a Ph.D., and took over the direction of the laboratory after Jacqueline's retirement. Gladys and her husband Gabe have been, and still are, close friends of Jacqueline's. Jacqueline finally became a professor at Baylor College of Medicine, because her work was internationally recognized, and the college received many requests for her promotion. As this was the most advanced academic rank she could not look for further achievements. She retired soon after because she wanted to paint, and because Baylor ceased contributing to her retirement funds.

Jacqueline also calculated that she would have more cash to spend if she retired without working. Having time and money, she then started to explore the world, and went on many organized trips in the company of Marie, a friend from Louisiana whom she met when Bob died. She also enjoyed the company of Dr. Tina Bangs who was a speech professor at the University of Texas and had an office near hers at TIRR for many years. She visited with Christian and Vincent Hepp, who moved from Houston to a small town in France, near Avignon. They traveled together to Venezuela and again to Russia and Uzbekistan, visiting the dream-like cities of Tashkent, Samarkand, and Bukhara. Jacqueline had a studio built in her house where she could have the space and the light to do oil painting. She took some painting courses at the school of the Fine Art Museum and also at the Art League of Houston. She packed her watercolors to paint wherever she went: Cannes, Nice, Brittany and Paris, Mexico, and Stamford, Connecticut, where she visited Simone. Jacqueline also enjoyed many trips organized by Elder Hostel, some in Texas, others in New Mexico.

At that time of her life she had a very pleasant neighbor, Lois, who was also a widow, and they shared small trips and local Texas outings. Unhappily, Lois was ill for a long time and died around 1985. Jacqueline also enjoyed the company of her old friend, Dr. Ilse Mannheimer, who lived across the street, and of her sister, Marga. Both died a long time ago. Jacqueline had to make new friends. She was lucky to meet Nicole, who was a friend of Christiane Hepp, and another younger woman, Christine. Both are French. She also had lasting friendship with Pat Schier, whom she met when Bob worked in real estate. Pat lives in Austin and visits often. She is very dynamic and has two daughters, one in college and the other working in Houston. Jacqueline has replaced the front lawn with a big garden, where most of the time there are enough roses to make flower arrangements to paint. She now has about five hundred paintings stored behind her garage where Bob had built a workshop. Jacqueline still uses the workshop to frame her paintings.

Some years later, Jacqueline had an awful mishap. She was hanging a diploma in the corridor when she fell and had to spend three months in a wheelchair. She managed her life with the help of her friends, and did all her rehabilitation in the pool and the hot tub in the backyard. A couple of years later, she couldn't walk, and she had to have surgery on her back. She fell again and had another operation. Again Jacqueline did all her rehabilitation in the pool and the hot tub, after being taught by a professional therapist who came several times to her home.

Age finally took its toll on her. Even though she had to stop playing tennis, Jacqueline is still relatively active and exercises daily in the pool and hot tub, for one hour. At eighty-nine, she still drives during the daytime, but seldom on freeways since she had cataract surgery on both eyes and has macular degeneration in one eye. She has no special interest in any man, though Seymour still calls and sends her birthday and Valentine's Day cards. She has an abundance of kindness and affection from Elisabeth and Jean Francois, and MT, as well as some faithful old friends. She takes pride in remembering her scientific accomplishments and knowing that her work benefited the paralyzed patients at TIRR. Jacqueline is also proud that her niece, Ann, has her own occupational therapy office in New Jersey, specializing in hand care, and that Alain, an architect, is now a well-known designer in New York City. Jacqueline has little spare time, still enjoying oil painting, cooking dinner for friends, and reading romantic novels!

As with all older people, Jacqueline started thinking about her past, and reminisced about her affair with her Vietnamese lover, Tuoc. She dug out his old letters, but she had a lot of difficulty reading and translating them to English. While reading these letters she was fascinated to realize how the past always stays in the memory regardless of how far people live from each other. These letters are a collection of hard-to-read scribbling, written on paper as thin as toilet paper. They were mailed from Vietnam in 1957, after Tuoc's departure from Paris, and twenty years later, after the war had ended. She reread and translated all the letters to find out if Tuoc's choice to return to communist Vietnam, and her choice to immigrate to the USA, had been wise, and to assess what both had gained and lost.

While Simone, Jean, Ann and Alain lived in Paris, they became very fond of the Vietnamese painter LePho, his wife, and their children. Jacqueline made sure her sister, and niece and nephew knew the origin of this friendship, to realize that she and Tuoc had known him during the Nazi occupation of France.

IX

Tuoc in Vietnam: Nineteen Letters to Jacqueline and Suzanne

Reading the letters from Tran Hu Tuoc, Jacqueline could appreciate the consequences of his decision to return to war-torn Vietnam and her decision not to marry him. It was only after a ten-year silence that some letters reached Jacqueline and her mother, Madame Claus. The letters were carried to East Germany, a Communist country then. From there a French friend and colleague of Tuoc's could mail them, either directly to the USA or, more often, to Madame Claus in Paris, who then forwarded the letters to her daughter!

The first letters that reached Jacqueline described the adventures of a 400-mile trip across the jungle, to Hanoi and the Democratic Republic of Vietnam around 1947. The next related Tuoc's first trip to France and his visits to Madame Claus in Paris. In his first letter to Jacqueline, he described his participation in the guerilla battles fought for the freedom of Vietnam, and he reminisced about his days with Jacqueline in Paris. Other letters contained more recollections of the past, together with descriptions of his professional achievements.

Tran Hu Tuoc was born in 1910 and educated in Hanoi, Vietnam, which was then a French colony. He was from a wealthy family, and at the age of nineteen, he went to Paris to attend medical school. Subsequently, he received specialized training as a surgeon for problems of the nose, ear and larynx (the specialty of Otorhinolaryngology, ORL), in children. The training was under the direction of Dr. Le Mee, a follower of the teachings of Dr. Chevalier Jackson, a pioneer of ORL in the USA. His training hospital was Necker Enfants Malades, a very old hospital built over a city block, consisting for the most part of many one-story stone buildings. This hospital was located at the corner of the rue de Vaugirard and the Boulevard de Montparnasse in Paris. He operated in the Blumenthal Pavilion, which was donated by the USA. Tuoc left France in 1947. After many years of hardship, he resumed the practice of pediatric ORL surgery in Hanoi, Vietnam, at a hospital called The Frontline. Later he became the Minister of Health of the Socialist Republic of Vietnam, and the Director of the Society of Otorhinolaryngology and Cervico-facial Pathology.

Some contact was made between the government of France and Vietnam in 1957, but it was only twenty years later, in 1977, that progress was achieved in the relationship between the countries. Tuoc was able to write letters in 1957 addressed to Jacqueline, his former fianceé, with whom he spent 1939 to 1941 in Paris. Two of these years (1939 and 1940) were in the above named hospital, where Jacqueline was an intern in pharmacy, and a jack-of-all-trades, while most of the male employees were fighting the war. Many of the letters were addressed to Jacqueline's mother, who lived on rue Scheffer, in Paris, and could forward them to Jacqueline. At the time, there was no mail between communist countries and the USA. Dr. Tran Hu Tuoc resumed writing to Jacqueline through her mother twenty years later, and continued from 1977 until 1983. He died from complications of prostate cancer in 1984, at about seventy-four years of age. Jacqueline learned of his death shortly after from their mutual friend, the painter LePho, who lived in Paris with his French wife Paulette and their children. The LePho family had become close friends with Suzanne, Simone, Jean, Annie and Alain, who all lived in Paris at the time.

Tuoc's letters are very sentimental about his relationship with Jacqueline and showed his nostalgia for the relatively happy years during the German occupation of Paris and the murderous Second World War. His descriptions of the re-birth of a medical community in Vietnam, which occurred with the help of physicians from former enemies such as France, and from communist countries, are fascinating. The group called Medecins sans Frontière, who took over such responsibilities, is active all over the world today. In the following letters, Tuoc's description of the specific injuries he treated in children such as burns caused by napalm and hearing damaged by frequent loud explosions, is especially interesting, as are the descriptions of the naked earth, devoid of vegetation in the war zones!

Tran Hu Tuoc
Hanoi

Hotel St. James
202 rue de Rivoli
Paris 1e

June 28, 1957

Dear Jacqueline,
    Since June I am officially delegated as a physician to Paris where I immediately telephoned rue Scheffer to have some news, and to take the time to have lunch with your mother, Madame Claus. Therefore I was able to get more detailed news. I am very pleased that you are successful and also in good health.
    These 10 years were filled by extraordinary events; I lived through much hardship, during which I learned a lot.
    Do you remember that we watched a movie "The Adventures of Dr. X"? I do not recall the name, but what we saw together does not compare with what I saw and went through. But it is so wonderful that I am now able to relate all of it.

We traveled a lot, then I nearly died. My belly was opened when I was only 95 pounds. Then we traveled another 400 miles by foot, in the jungle, in a tropical rain forest and I was always alone, loaded with work.

Only now was I reunited with my friends and my family and I was named the head of the laryngology department in the hospital "Le Frontline." I work there 14 to 16 hours daily. My friends and relatives didn't find me different from when I left for France, at age 19—still very phlegmatic.

My visit with you and with Madame Claus at the end of my stay in Paris gave me another joy. Professionally the trip gave me a chance to participate in meetings and a small reception aimed to re-establish the relations between France and the Democratic Republic of Vietnam. These events gave me an opportunity to travel to Paris. I would have liked to exchange more words . . .

Believe always in my deep affection and true friendship and allow me to send you my kisses.

Affectionately,
Tran Hu Tuoc

P.S. I am leaving July 2 for Berlin, Ryn, Menon, Peking, and Hanoi.

Tran Hu Tuoc
Hanoi, Professor a la Faculteé de Medecine
Republique Democratique DO Vietnam

Hotel St. James
200 rue de Rivoli
Paris, 7e

August 28, 1957

My dear Jacqueline,

It took me forever to answer your letter, only because I lack the time and when I had a chance to start, my thinking was interrupted so I gave up! But believe me, this last year, I thought of you a lot, many times: strange, is it not!

Today is August 28, 1957: what are you doing at this hour this day? I am on vacation in a resort at an altitude of about 3000 feet, nearly alone, with only a few friends. Therefore I am recalling memories from the apartment on rue Blomet and our lives.

I cannot resist the temptation to chat with you a little . . . excuse me if my French is incorrect, but I lack practice, besides, now your poor friend speaks other languages and sometimes even writes poems in Chinese. You asked me what I did during the last 10 years—how can I tell you? I was in barricades in Hanoi; I participated with the guerillas and brought a modest share to the liberation of my country, tasted the intoxicating joy of victory, endured the hardest deprivations during the "resistance" as every one did . . . and now I am submerged by loads of work to organize the return of peace after so many years of war.

And our country is not yet unified. Since 1947 my life had only one aim . . . and I nearly lost my life several times to achieve it . . . which helped me to reach serenity (or wisdom) to measure everything to its true value.

Believe me, dear Jacqueline, in life one must always pay, and often very dearly. And the remembrances of youth are like oases, which occur less and less. And now, in the middle of my life I can say that life is a strange thing, and happiness, even inside, is such a relative happening, whereas living intensely is so much richer. It is not only more fecund for a brain thirsty for knowledge and understanding.

Apart from general events, you cannot imagine in what extraordinary conditions I operated in surgery all these years . . . to end up being operated on myself in a dramatic one. Finally we were able to create a Laryngology Department where in 1955 I became the Chairman, so you can see I am being faithful to my first love.

Speaking of love, I can assure you truthfully that I led the life of a Trappist monk, because with the peripatetic life I had, and the incertitude of the future I could not give up my freedom and get married. Of course occasional visions of tenderness and stability appeared every now and then . . . but faithful to some memories my mind does not succeed to reach a solution and I continue to live alone, burdened by the workload and by the heat. All this without any merit, if there is merit, this country is of such Puritanism! Maybe this will change, I still ignore it because it depends on many factors.

Actually I am still at the Medical Faculty, Chief of Service, Director of the largest hospital of the extreme Orient and the President of the Medical Society of Vietnam, adviser, and so on. . . .

You see, dear Jacqueline, I don't have the time to plant the flowers that you love! I don't know if I have changed, but while I write, I feel again like the very young man while he watered the geraniums, with my hand stained with the soil lifted in boxes on a sunny balcony, which means a respite in my life and an instant of happiness. I wanted in June to replant my geraniums, but could not do it! Oh, if I could send you from here the magnificent orchids which at 3000 feet are all over the mountains. I wanted so much to send these tropical plants with such wonderful shapes and colors, slimness in the shape and sweetness of shades and such elegance in their outline. Jacqueline, will you ever know these blooms, which enrapture me during my hours of solitude?

Did I tell you that I adopted a tiny young girl who got married and that I am now a grandfather? How soft are the arms of the children around the neck when they call you grandfather.

Alas, the grandchildren are very far away because their parents hold a diplomatic job in a foreign country. I still have my old mother, nearly 80 years old, who watches over me as if I were a 19-year-old boy, the age when I left her.

I will be so happy to get a letter from you. I think you are already married to this noble Irishman and that you now have a handsome baby, to the great joy of Simone and of your parents to whom I will write in Paris. Keep in good health and write to me.

Very affectionately,
Tran Hu Tuoc

Paris, France

July 14, 1977

Dear Madame Claus,

I am so happy to have your letter. I called by telephone. I could only join Rosa who told me that you had left and that you are well again to be able to travel. Looking at your writing I know that you are in good shape: you will live to be a hundred!

I am heartbroken for Jacqueline; please convey to her most affectionate thoughts. She can write me: Institute National ORL, Hanoi RSVN, and the letter will reach me. (ORL, Otorhinolar-gyngology?—RSVN—Republic Sovietique du Vietnam.)

After Paris we are joining a congress in Berlin, then Hanoi. Lots of work, mostly now after 30 years of war. Lots of courage and stubbornness were needed after these terrible years. Finally, freedom and independence for our children and grandchildren. I will try to take the time to write to Jacqueline. Tell her lot of things: it was our youth, our illusions, our hopes. I have also fond memories of Simone and her husband.

At my next trip I do hope to see you in better health.

I kiss you affectionately.

Can you give me Jacqueline's address? I will write her in Houston.

Tran Hu Tuoc

Tran Hu Tuoc—Hanoi

Hemingdorf, Germany

August 19, 1977
Institut National d'ORL
Bach Mai, Hanoi

Dear Madame Claus,
    We are spending our vacations in the Democratic Republic (Germany) (RDA) for one month and I think about you. I am so happy to read your letters—only looking at your writing, so young and firm: your health is excellent.
    The most precious memories are those I have from you, these years are perhaps the most profound and moving.
    Tell Jacqueline that I think of her often, and of her recent loss. Did it affect her deeply—is her morale still superb?
    Soon I will return to work. At the end of September I probably will visit you in Paris—there is still so much work . . .
    I wish you better health, a long life. Over a hundred! (Even without the complete address your letters always reach me.)

                    Very affectionately,
                    Tran Hu Tuoc

Viet Nam ban Chu Cong Hoa
Doc lop Tu do Houb phuc
Ha Noi, ngay

September 2, 1977

Dear Jacqueline,
    Returning from a vacation in the Republique Democratique Allemande (RDA) on the Baltic Sea, I am very moved to find your letter in my mail. Already I received a letter from your mother where I learned the event [the sudden death of

Bob] and I never had such a feeling of helplessness to grab me . . . and you must feel it in all your heart. I understand all your feelings!

It is nice for you to develop a taste for the trees and the birds. The many years that we spent in the jungle were the most wonderful . . . so many orchids . . . oh, if I could possibly send you at least one between the sheets of paper.

Dr. Yves Cachin had to leave the research work for which he is passionate. After 30 years we are maintaining a network between laryngologists in all the Vietnamese country, North and South, but it is still short of our needs for 5 million residents.

In Hanoi, since 1966, we have a National Institute of Otorhinolargyngology, that does partly clinical work and partly research on immunology and treatments of the cancers of the pharynx and the larynx, the pituitary and others. For your information, I still do 4 to 5 hours a day of surgery, then lectures, research, and so on! Alas, there is no time to read a good book and shut off the work, to live for one's self.

Did you know that in 1972 three-fourths of the personnel of my Institute were detained in Bach May by B52 bombing? That time I nearly did not make it. Luckily the patients were evacuated, but we lost 28 medical doctors, nurses, interns, only in our Institute. We reconstructed. I took many trips to Europe and Paris to recruit medical personnel. Now we have a whole department for children.

Several years ago, because of the war and the numerous explosions, there was a need to treat injuries of the middle and internal ear. The damages from 30 years of war are horrible. You cannot imagine the effect of the toxic gases, and the napalm burns. There are no insects, no birds, moonscape-like land. One must have seen all of that to understand how savage and barbarous men can be with their improved war technology.

Be sure that in your faraway corner, you have someone who thinks about you . . . and if there is some telepathy you must have buzzing in your ears.

Recently, from Berlin, I wrote again to Madame Claus. I admire her energy: her writing is marvelous by its steadiness and elegance.

Now, with communications getting increasingly normal, maybe we can write each other more frequently. At the end of September I will be in Paris, then in London, and perhaps at the end of the year I could see you in your home!

I am always dreaming and hoping. I feel well; I walk six miles each day in a big park. I row a canoe, and so on.

I rush, the mail is picked up. . . . See you soon.

> I kiss you very affectionately.
> Tran Hu Tuoc

Look at the paper with the letterhead from our Medical Institute in Hanoi.

Hotel Sofitel Bourbon
32, Rue St. Dominique, 75007 Paris
Tel 555 21 11 Telex 25019

November 11, 1977

Dear Madame Claus,

I am on a mission for a few days in Paris. I called your home several times but there was no answer. I was downhearted.

Lately I am traveling a lot; it is very tiring but it is necessary for the country for its reconstruction after thirty years of war.

I bid you excellent health and a long life.

> Very affectionately,
> Tran Hu Tuoc

April 20, 1978

My dear Jacqueline,

Your letter from January 3, 1978, arrived on March 25, 1978. You cannot imagine the strange feeling of fulfillment, of hope and of deep affection that it resurrected in me! It is so good to have someone dear to whom I can talk about everything from so far! I will ask Dr. Yves Cachin who is coming to visit me to bring this letter—this way may be faster because between the Vietnam and the USA there are still postal problems, among others. Also, I think it is possible to invite you as a cultural guest? Anyway, I am less worried after reading your letter. I found that you are in good health, with several viewpoints, and we are closer to each other than we believe. You were right to take life positively, and for some things you are less favored than me . . . all said without bitterness.

These days I begin to understand life and feel more inner peace for which I am greatly thankful to you . . . one could reminisce. You could not live the way I have to live to merit the freedom and independence which I missed when we met. Finally I could not offer you the support. One pays for everything in the world, because if you recall I already told you, "Vanita vanitas," so it is.

In June I received a short letter of Madame Claus, charming, really at her age so lively and present. I always admire her affectionately.

You know that lately I went all over the world, far too much for my taste. Now that you have a friend who reads Chinese, ask her to read those few pages from Toucan, the great poet of the Tang dynasty.

After such reading you will know my latest mood. I extensively study foreign languages and love to do it. Do you know that I still practice medicine and surgery, because even now there are still, due to the war, many cancers of the thyroid and of the hypothalamus? We have an operating technique that gives good results. Our Institute has a laboratory for chemical research and it comes to my mind, since 1946 I never operated as much. In 20 years my personal operating statistic is 220 brain and cerebellum abscesses. We have not worked further than the infection stage. And as we are in a country in the developing phase, one must think about preventive medicine. Therefore, from the working viewpoint it is terrible and it occupies my time all-day and part of the night. Without such preoccupations can you imagine the remembrances overcoming the dreamer that I remain!

From your letter I can see that you remain very busy. If by chance I reach the USA I will do what is needed to pay you a visit: will you agree? I have a small cottage in the middle of Hanoi, given to me very recently because I am 68 years of age . . . and marvelous thing, after 30 years, I have my own bedroom, for me alone and my books and it is so good. And when I close the key I shut out the outside world, and "vive the liberty." In 1977 the government invited me for four weeks in Paris . . . but I could only stand three weeks and spent the vacation in RDA [Republic Democratic Allemande]. Nevertheless, I do not believe that we have all we need. I can tell you that we still lack many things. The Vietnamese regime is good to those above sixty years old. So I have good health and I regret that we cannot take walks together. I love to walk and each day I try to do it regularly, at least two to three miles, but the air in Hanoi in reconstruction is so dusty that it takes away some of the pleasure. I also have a dog, a mountain race, which is very attached to me. Each evening he waits for me and gives me his paw for a friendly shake.

Thanks for the petunias and geraniums that you planted. I would like to help you. I was rather good, I admit, as you may recall. I only have a small square of garden, where I also tried to grow geraniums. They don't do well, it is too hot and too humid, and sometimes I dream of a fireplace, like at the Enfant Malades Hospital intern quarters and of a chimney fire in winter when in the evening one shivers of cold. I will ask Dr. Yves Cachin, the big boss of Villejuif Hospital where I sent one of my assistants to work in 1977, to send you a souvenir from Hanoi, but I do not know what you prefer: a necklace, a pendant, or something for Toto! It is too bad that you have no children, they can be loved selfishly as you said, though they escape from the day they are born.

My daughter is 19 years old, in the third year of medical school. She is rather tall and pleasant. I will mail you a picture if it becomes possible. In 1966, the year of the most atrocious bombings of Vietnam, we had a boy who was 12 years old on December 26, 1972. That year both of us nearly died, victims of the bombings.

We still miss the foreign medical journals. Perhaps some day you can send me some American journals and your publications. It would be wonderful. Have you carried out your plan to travel to Asia? One day you will go swimming in the Bay of Along, the eighth marvel of the world. I am going there in April with Dr. Yves Cachin.

I must admit that I love the sea, and every year I often stay whole days on the beach, either working or dreaming. You should come when you stop working! Do you ever have a time for retirement in the USA? Here we work until exhaustion, mostly for the responsible leaders. In 1976 we had a television documentary on our Institute, which was seen in Paris—I am still photogenic!

Last June I was able to call Rosa, as well as other French friends. By the way, how are Simone and Jean? I stopped because my pigeons were noisy at the window, begging for food! Do you have birds? They are wonderful to watch playing. We also have a cat, mostly friendly with my daughter but he is greedy and fat. I am not fond of him. I prefer those in need. How is your ankle? How is it that you have always been wearing spiked heels? By the way, do you get your clothing in Paris or Houston? Is there a difference between the fashions in both countries? What is your current taste in clothing? Do you still have the habit to pull on your cuticles when you are in a quandary or embarrassed? Give me news of your uncle Jean Alexandre, who is the president of the Violet Perfumery. Many things to catch up in 32 years—one's life goes on but suddenly our age has changed. . . .

July 20, 1978

It is when one reaches the age when besides work there is time for remembering faithful friends and to speculate on the future, to become detached from many things—fresh air, birds, flowers and friends are more important. A friend is leaving for Paris and will deliver this letter to Madame Claus who is kind enough to mail it to you. Our mail service is not yet reliable.

                                        I think of you very affectionately,
                                        Tran Hu Tuoc

Hanoi

May 13, 1978

My dear Jacqueline,
    A friend from the Hopital Necker, Dr. Yves Cachin, came with me to the Bay of Along, and surrounded by a lavish landscape, we talked about you. It was an official visit to Vietnam for only one week. See: life is full of the unknown and surprises! I will not be astounded if very soon you will come to Hanoi or I will come to Houston—one should never give up! Did you get the letter I mailed to rue Scheffer, to be sure it will reach you? Did you travel as planned? How did you like southeast Asia? Write a lengthy letter if you have the time. I give a kiss to Toto (the dog) that I already like, because I have a very similar one.
    So much time since we have seen each other, even for a few days, a long friendship.
    I use this opportunity to mail you a photograph of the Baie d'Along, Dr. Yves Cachin and my other colleagues. Have you changed much?
    This is only a short letter because I must give it to Yves, the "letter carrier" toward the city of Paris.

                                        Very affectionately,
                                        Tran Hu Tuoc

Bo Y Te
Vien Tai-Mui-Hong
Viet Nam Dan Chu Cong Hoa
Doc lap-Tu-do-Hanh phuc
Hanoi, ngay

August 19, 1978

Dear Madame Claus,
    I had fresh news of you from Jacqueline. I was pleased to
know that you feel in great shape—try to become a centenarian*.
Your writing and your style tell me that you will joyfully go over
100 years.
    We love you with affection and I think of you often.

                        Accept my best wishes,
                        Yours,
                        Tran Hu Tuoc

P.S. Can you do me the favor to forward this letter to Jacqueline? Thanks.

Republique Socialiste du Viet Nam
Ministère de la Santé
Institut d'ORL
Hanoi

August 19, 1978

Dear Jacqueline,
    I just received your letter, and the huge pleasure it gave
me makes me delay my answer. It is true, the reason my writing
is not very legible is that I had so much to write. But you are

---

* Suzanne almost made it! She died at age 97.

101

not aware of my efforts to make my scribblings legible . . . the problem is probably also due to the fact that you are used to reading English. Jacqueline, you still have the same spelling errors. It makes me feel younger.

I asked how you dressed in order to imagine what you feel, because my clothing worries have been reduced to nothing for so many years! My only passion is the sea! Often I catch the slightest opportunity to escape toward the seaside! The Vietnam has more than 1800 miles of coastal land—I would love it if some day you could stretch your body into the Pacific surf. I just returned from spending three weeks in the South: the water is wonderful, clear and cool, with moderate waves, and the beach sand is soft, white, fine and marvelous in several places. I am back with a suntan just like a true fisherman! There, a day without eyeglasses and wearing a tiny slip, I was mistaken for the boss of a "jonques" company. You see my mental and corporeal dispositions!

And the nights of full moon, how delicious it is to bathe in the pale gold of the waves full of phosphorescence. I would love if you could at least one time come to Vietnam, so you could understand me a little more and know me better!

I hope your trip in September has given you some better knowledge of the portion of the world that suffers acutely of being under developed. Vietnam has been in a state of war for over 30 years and is hardly reunited; it is still undergoing lots of shortages and enormous suffering.

Dear Jacqueline, can you imagine that at my age I do not have enough sugar and lemons: I thought of these because you liked lemonades. But if you don't take refreshments, it is fine. Often this kind of thinking helps us overcome everything. I had a chance to get detached from so much among such miseries and injustices, and a huge love for freedom and independence. Everything is vanity and vanity!

It is true that we always remain children at heart, which helps us to look at life with a very personal viewpoint.

You gave me a complete list of our friends: LePho the painter is a man without ideals, or in other words, with a frivolous ideal—he sided with our enemy Bao Dai and cut off his relations with us. He denied that he owed me money. When I left in 1947 he signed a promissory note to cash bad checks and late fees. Later I learned that the wealthy do not like to pay their debts. Vu Cao Dam is a talented painter, I learned from his wife Reneé that he is in poor health. I also learned that many do not like to remember the bad times they went through. I had given a lot of financial help to Vu Cao Dam, when no one purchased his paintings. But later Reneé refused even to see any Vietnamese people.

If you have a chance, you should read "The Voyage of Monsieur Bernichon" from Labiche, it will help you understand better those poor souls who think they live well when in reality they live miserably, even submerged in abundance, because their life is so confined. Alas, so many great and beautiful things are available if you can consecrate your life for it . . . give away all you have without any hope to succeed, in exchange for whatever it could be.

Maybe some day I will describe these years when my life hung on a thread always ready to break! Now I keep myself in good shape: I still do surgery, I teach, carry on research on the cancer of the hypothalamus, which occurs frequently among us, in contrast with Europe where there is a greater incidence of laryngeal cancers. I study the evolutionary history of the conventional specialty of Otorhinolaryngology (ORL), and have begun to study also traditional medicines to assess what they bring to the ORL specialty. Unhappily our neighbors in the North are still aggressive, but we will eventually win!

How is Madame Claus? I love and admire such strength at her age, her writing reflects her vitality. Simone must be very happy. I saw Rosa and Marc, always young and charming. Rosa always smiling, and it reminded me of the evening not long ago when you were also there . . . and you pulled the cuticles of your fingernails, keeping your old habit. In Rosa's house and garden I used to be able to relax, but could not any more. Tell Rosa that I have no opportunity to relax and let go of our worries and be sociable and that the moments spent in her garden are my fondest and most alive memories from overseas.

I do understand why you do not recall Yves Cachin who was an intern at Dr. Le Mee's after I became Dr. Le Mee's assistant. It was the year after Dr. Bauke was jailed by the Germans that Dr. Yves Cachin came to intern at Dr. Le Mee's at Necker Enfants Malades Hospital. Yves was very moved when we were reunited in Vietnam after being apart thirty years! He was greatly impressed by our achievements in Public Health in the Provinces, the districts and the communes and if you could guess what we gave to build all of it, starting from zero, especially for the ORL.

Please write me, so I do not forget French. I think of you with much affection, like the limpid hours of our youth.

Tran Hu Tuoc

Dresden
May 9, 1979

My dear Jacqueline,

You can see that my life is such that I returned from the front against the Chinese in good health . . . and now I have an enormous prostate and a high fever for the last five days. Therefore I was shipped as an emergency to the RDA [Republic Democratic of Allemagne] for rest and fun. I feel much better except for the food which for us Vietnamese is nearly inedible. But the friendliness of the Socialists helps to withstand all things.

The Committee of the French Communism invited me to come to Paris and France! But I think I will not accept the invitation: there is nothing good about returning to the places where life gave us something!

How are you? We were invited to the USA: our National Institute of ORL was filmed and we were interviewed for a long time. I said the Vietnam population does not hold a grudge against the people of America, though the devastation due to the use of various gases by the U.S. is still there! And it incites the hatred of the poor ignorant and despicable Chinese. Do not worry, but I nearly died recently while visiting the frontiers. But you know, my dear Jacqueline, my fate is like the meal of the condemned, to live a long time to see many things! It is sometimes tiring, but it is entertaining!

You did not talk about your trip to southeast Asia.

Maybe this year I will make up my mind to come to the USA. But this means a life of luxury, therefore I am searching for dollars, and Le Pho is on the other political side . . . always pleasant but so selfish; Mai Thu has no money; Vu Cao Dam is bossed by his wife. Therefore, last year I was invited by a French association for four weeks, but could only afford three. Among so many people who did not experience our miseries they want organized projects. Life is so strange, sometimes, to feel better, I hold my breath!

What are you doing? Even at my age I walk fast and for a long time, two to four miles a day. Therefore, be careful, if I come to Houston, which I know well, from books of course; we will run a marathon.

Here we have beautiful orchids that I would like to send you, but this is difficult, therefore I can only send you the perfume of these living blooms which I love. Now that I live in a free and independent Vietnam I can write freely which I could not do when colonization made us silent! You could not know what it was like when we had no freedom, no independence.

In East Germany the population is kind to the Vietnamese because we defeated Imperialism.

I visited museums in Dresden (it reminded me of our meeting at the Chagall exhibit in Paris) where there are many quattrocento, a few impressionists, some Van Gogh. I did admire some very good Guillaumins and Pissarros . . . during these moments I wished you to be present, to be together and share our impressions. But this is life: one must always pay, and dearly, very dearly, to be happy . . . or only to have peace of mind. Alas, so it is.

What are you doing this minute? Right now I am tired of wandering here and there. I would like to lie down next to the sea, look at the waves, the ever-changing colors of the tropical seas, and sleep in the evenings. Do you remember the verses of Michelangelo, "it is so sweet to sleep, sweeter to be made of stone"? As we can't be made of stone we should sleep. Well, three or four hours of sleep is a dream of a gift!

Since yesterday we have had magnificent sunshine and I am sending a little piece of that sun in memory of our young years together. We also have lilacs not yet in bloom. I am trying very hard to return on March 20th to Vietnam. My dear Jacqueline, if you could imagine all the work I have had, have, and will have. My work helps me stop the memories of the past. I am writing a book of Vietnam, the history of medicine and of otorhinolaryngology, and at the beginning of September there is a new chairmanship of the History of Medicine at the Hanoi Faculty. As you see, Jacqueline, I accumulate many projects, in order to avoid thinking!

I am always looking forward to your letters. With a correct address they will reach me with a lengthy delay, but they arrive!

Really, Mme Claus is splendid. Her handwriting is still neat and vigorous. I was sorry not to be able to call her on the phone, but I was there at four in the morning.

Keep in good health—try to laugh heartily as you are still very young in my memory.

Very affectionately,
Tran Hu Tuoc

Société Vietnamienne
D'oto-Rhino-Laryngologie Et
De Pathologie Cervico-Faciale
Le Comité De Direction
République Socialiste Du V.N.

Dresden
May 19, 1979

My dear Jacqueline,

When you receive this note I will already be far from Dresden, from the RDA, where, I don't know.

I looked since the first burst of lilac blooms for one with five petals to send you, but alas I could not find any, therefore I send three petals . . . not blue, but white . . . hoping that you do not have to pay for all the flowers that I could not send for such a long time.

My health is much better—at my age I have all the privileges of the cardiac patients even if I am not one, I only have a small inflammation of the prostate.

Keep healthy, send me news to Hanoi, ORL Institute is enough.

I do not know when I will go to the USA. Anyway I will call you on the phone.

Very affectionately,
Tran Hu Tuoc

P.S. I hope I will not be censored from here because of the flowers?

Société Vietnamienne
D'oto-Rhino-Laryngologie Et
De Pathologie Cervico-Faciale
Le Comité de Direction
République Socialiste Du V.N.

Berlin

December 1, 1979

Dear Jacqueline,

Already December, and soon Christmas and the cold and the snow. How are you? Well, I hope.

I am here for some days in Europe for an ORL congress.

I write you because I wanted to send you a large pine tree for Christmas, but I was told it was impossible. I will try to do something. I don't know what yet. How is your work and your health? Write to me! I am in great shape. I always hope. I am so busy with my new chairmanship in the History of Medicine and the chair and the ORL Institute to direct. As you, I did not waste any time, but there are improvements, allowing me to dream of other things.

If I stay a while in RDA I will write to Mme Claus, of whom I am so very fond. Is she still in good shape? For her age she writes beautifully.

What is new with you and your friends?

Unhappily we are still busy fighting. Recently I was on the frontier. It was interesting as we had a peaceful dinner under an alert.

Do you have white hair? I have many; it looks very nice when I am at professional meetings. I have been invited to go to the Academy in Dresden. I am sure I will go, even if Dresden does not have much attraction for me.

Ah, finally I have a piano. Not a great piano, nearly straight but I spend some time to redo a little music: Brahms, do you believe?

What are you doing for Christmas? And the other Christmases? Finally life goes by, and it is strange, don't you believe?

Well, from the bottom of my heart I wish you peace, perhaps happiness.

I kiss you with much affection.

Merry Christmas and my best wishes for a happy new year.

Write to me,
Tran Hu Tuoc

Tran Huo Tuoc
Hanoi

Berlin

December 22, 1979

Dear Jacqueline,

The day after tomorrow I will take a plane from Berlin to Hanoi, twenty hours of flying and today I am writing to you because here we are in the middle of the Christmas season and everywhere there are toys and flowers. I tried to ship some to you but it is not possible: too far! Therefore, you should be satisfied with these few lines of writing which will stay longer on the paper than barely opened flower buds.

Have you received the few lines of writing hastily sketched from Dresden? We attended a symposium in Dresden at their Academy, then I will stay in Berlin a full week. Finally we have the OK for December 23 for a plane going to Vietnam with only one stop in Karachi!

How are you? Do you still swim? Are you in good shape? Is anybody courting you with offhanded charm, American style! There, are people still kissing on the mouth . . . or the cheek?

This year I am invited to Paris, but I must admit that Paris is no longer a temptation because for a long time now I can't allow myself to search for shadows that are lost or misplaced.

Ah, I will have many things to tell you because when I think about it, what I was able to see and to hear, all around the world during the last thirty and some years would make you laugh or smile and perhaps also, exhale!

Anyway, I am in good health, even better and better, which bothers me a little because I am given so much work. Every week I operate two or three times, mainly for cancers of the hypopharynx. I demand that my young assistant learn English and I make great efforts toward technical improvement. And it was found, alas, that this was not enough, and I was given a new chairmanship for the History of Medicine, so I have to read again in Greek and Latin.

Ah, this year I finished writing two books, one in French on a new technique for operating on pharyngeal and laryngeal cancers, and another book in Vietnamese on the History of Medicine. I will try to send you a copy. And at the Hanoi Congress of Medicine I was also asked to write my memories of our President. I wait for your letters. They finally reach me, with a delay, but they do reach me.

Dear Jacqueline, Noel brings to me all memories, but alas, I am stopping. Imagine that I send you many flowers with much affection and friendship.

And when I write to you I may perhaps console myself with many things! During our life maybe one can never reach happiness . . . perhaps happiness is only a dream. Instead, one feels peace in the accomplishment of a goal and, as "Le Loup" from Vigny, one can fade discreetly with the unforgettable smile of Buddha that I know you saw in the pagodas in Java and all Shintoist temples of Japan.

I kiss you very affectionately and wish you a very nice Christmas: you will feel a very light wind which is the moving tenderness of a deep friendship. I think of you often at the other end of the world.

Merry Christmas, lots of luck, and better health for 1980 . . . and maybe we can meet again.

110

If you write to Rosa and Marc, tell them about my peregrinations. (I do not have their address) but I will write to Madame Claus.

Tran Hu Tuoc

Tran Hu Tuoc
Hanoi

Berlin

December 22, 1979

Dear Madame Claus,
I am spending one month in the Republic Democratic Allemande, for an important otorhinolaryngology congress and several other symposiums, and we will take a KLM plane tomorrow for Hanoi.
It is Christmas, I think of Paris, of you, and I send you my very affectionate thoughts and my best wishes for better health next year.
Did you have a pleasant Christmas? I just wrote to Jacqueline but have no answer yet. And also I travel too much. In the Hanoi Medical School a new chair was created for the History of Medicine, and I am the first chairman. As you see, in Hanoi, in charge of two chairmanships I have little time for myself, often traveling, waiting for airplanes we can try to route. . . .
Believe, dear Madame Claus, in my affectionate fidelity and receive my sincere wishes for Christmas and New Year.

Tran Hu Tuoc

Tran Hu Tuoc
Hanoi

June 21, 1981

My dear Jacqueline,

Even though your letter arrived two months late, it filled me with pleasure. I find again the dear Jacqueline with all her spelling errors, enormous for the purist that I am! I finally find you again! I regretted not having written to your mother.

Yes, I went around a lot, as you will tell me again. I had the chance to see nearby countries and also further away where I have given lectures . . . and so on . . .

I always hope, so you will understand . . . two books, one on the history of occidental medicine and the other on the history of ORL, and a monograph in French, yes, on laryngeal cancers in Vietnam, describing a new surgical technology. At the end of this month I will try to send it to you [the monograph] because as I know you do not yet read Vietnamese. Too bad!

You are lucky to eat Vietnamese dishes in the USA. Are these as well cooked as those prepared in the past in Paris? I have the habit to swim 2–3 times daily, it really helps to stay in good shape, there is nothing like it. I now walk six miles every day, not jogging but rapid walking, on the seashore. What a shame that I cannot yet invite you to come admire our coastal landscapes, so picturesque with the limpid water, and so healthy. These later years, it is the sea that gives me comfort and pleasure and I go as much as possible. My fingers are still steady, and I still attempt to do something to help hopeless patients. I hope to keep a long time this steadfastness, though as you recall I am getting close to my sixty-eighth year—I will be seventy in two years.*

There is a lot of work carried out in our institute, with six operating rooms with television on site and a good research

---

* Tuoc said in previous letters that he was born in 1910; therefore he should be 71 years of age! Here, he states that his birth was in 1913.

laboratory. You never told me your specialty? You could have helped in my work! I admire Madame Claus, at her age, to take such long trips. What vitality—I would like to have it when I am her age. And you, my dear, will you have such dynamism/I hope so for you. Poor Marc, how old is he, he has the radiation illness—and Rosa? Please write them on my behalf as I keep a wonderful memory of Choisy during those war years. Are Simone and Jean well? Can you tell them that I think about them. News broadcasts have a long delay, but news eventually reaches us.

Also, Mai Thu, the painter died from a cerebral hemorrhage last October, after having a successful exhibit. Le Pho, the one who did not worry, is still in good health. Vu Cao Dam is very diminished by illness. Finally, there is nothing to do about aging: the main thing is to stay young mentally and affectively, if possible!

You are lazy, because it is easier to send letters from where you live than from here to Texas . . . books, also. Let us try to stay in touch because one lives through the past toward the future. Lots of work, it helps to keep me in shape, and I am not losing the hope to see you again some day! Write to me, your letters always reach me and fill me with deep pleasure . . . even the misspellings give me joy each time I read your letter over again. You have not changed, me either. Embrace your friends for me . . . and I wish you lots of pleasure and happiness.

Yours affectionately,
Tran Hu Tuoc

P.S. Do you still have the habit to pull on the cuticles of your finger? Answer, please.

Bo Y Té
Vien-Tai-Mut Hong

Adams Hotel
3 rue de l'Odeon
Paris 325.90.6.7

December 11, 1982

Dear Madame Claus,
    I just arrived in Paris for a scientific mission, lasting several weeks. I hope you are in good health. Your last letter pleased me so much, your style and your writing are those of a young woman!
    Do you have news of Jacqueline? I will try to write her as soon as possible because in Paris, life is so busy.
    My best wishes for your good health, dear Madame.

                                        Very affectionately,
                                        Tran Hu Tuoc

Bay of Along
Vietnam

July 6, 1983

Dear Jacqueline,
    I do not know when you will receive this wave of energy pushing me to take a pen and write to you, in a period of total relaxation while I am looking at this marvelous Bay of Along where I wanted you to visit. But the fates said otherwise . . . though I don't give up because life is full of surprises. As soon as I got your last letter I sent a telegram to Madame Claus for her 95th birthday. My septuagenarian efforts to write legibly with my poor eyes make me tired!
    Yes, this year I reached seventy years old. I was very surprised to have reached that age! Yes, sometimes one needs to

stop and look behind and recall past events and glance towards the meaning of life . . . yes, these are not big words, at any age, I consider mine with surprise because I feel very young as I felt in the past—yes!

An unconscious, powerful strength helped me and directed me since my early youth. You will never know the mentality of a person that was brought into the world frustrated by lacking the most precious gift of life: freedom and independence! You mentioned in your last letter that there are now Vietnamese in Texas, though in 1940 you did not know I was Vietnamese. Thinking about it I smile now, and I can tell you that I did everything possible to have a modest part in the rebirth of Vietnam.

I read over your letter. Well, I did not, like you did, dream of helping the human race, though I only achieved my part, to become a truly free human, with a country. You were lucky not to be under the colonial regime, but for a while you jumped into the hell of the Nazi regime. I shared your feelings, and also of those with haunted eyes which had lost any human look. . . . Therefore, in order not to live in these conditions, during the last forty years I withstood with patience many hardships which return honor and serenity to those who have spent years to serve . . . this is all!

I will not speak about my physical condition, when I looked like a skeleton in 1951 . . . or the inferno of the bombs from B52s in 1970, or of being in the eye of the cyclone when I lived with unforgettable minutes, in the mist of my native country, which was three-fourths annihilated. Finally, we overcame all that. In 1982, my prostate was removed and also the descending colon (down with colon-ianism . . . sorry pun, right?) I recovered well. I walk three miles daily and am getting younger!

If you want to read an article in a French periodical regarding your old friend, look for the February issue (1983) (26) I believe of "The Generalist,"—there is a summary of my accomplishments.

You advise me to take some leisure, stop performing surgery, and give no more lectures. Alas, I have the habit, not the obligation, because already my students have accomplished a lot but, you know, I am a surgeon: faced with a catastrophic case I cannot stay quiet. Very recently I operated for two hours on a patient with an abscess of the cerebellum. I also gave four lectures of ORL in Gerontology.

My fingers did not shake, nor did my feet, and in the smothered silence of operating rooms I lived again the hours spent in the Pavilion Le Mee [Blumenthal] or the anguished minutes when we operated during the bombings. One does not escape his destiny. I am solidly planted on the ground of my country but now and then I think of Paris, of Choisy le Roi, of Rosa, so understanding with Marc . . . who allowed me to relax in their garden. The last time I was in Paris, I was too occupied by the workload to meet them, but I often thought affectionately of them and all of you, memories of my unstable, shaky youth.

I stop a while, the water of the gulf is pleasant today and I will take a dip, alone in my favorite laguna . . . see you soon.

To replace happiness which I could not aspire for, at least I reached a separate temporal peace with myself . . . which I think represents a lot! You contributed to it, I am thankful to you from the bottom of my heart and I will reach the turning point of my seventieth birthday with serenity, though still unsatisfied!

I have a twenty-four-year-old daughter who studies medicine with Dr. Yves Cachin, in Paris. Maybe she will take the opportunity to write you, or to see you. Help her a little, if you can. I also have a sixteen-year-old son who, after his baccalaureate, will enter the competitive examination for Les Grandes Ecoles. He is very handsome, already nearly taller than me . . . he is like the little Tuoc, at his age of expatriation in 1931.

Subsequently I will try to have a more regular correspondence with you . . . and I would like news from you for your birthday.

Very affectionately,
Tran Hu Tuoc

P.S. I will use the return of a friend to Paris to send this letter. I spent two marvelous months at the seaside, I am becoming desiccated and brown as an old sea wolf. I am shipping the puff of a thyphon.

Tran Hu Tuoc
Hanoi

l'Odeon Hotel
3 rue de l'Odéon
Paris 75006

October 25, 1983

My dear Jacqueline,

I am again in Paris, nearly against my will, because Dr. Yves Cachin, whom you know, could not come to Hanoi to attend a symposium on nasopharyngeal cancer (NPC) to be held between scientists and Vietnamese physicians in April 1983, which I am to coordinate! We have published much research work, but we have unhappily too many patients in such category.

How are you? Do you still work or are you reading? I have written to Madame Claus to ask how she was, if I have time I will certainly go visit her, as I love her dearly. But you know, in Paris and also Hanoi, I am overloaded with work. There is too much to do after more than thirty years of war! There are so many damages to repair, but we are doing everything possible to ameliorate the patient' status.

In July 1981 I was in Budapest for the 12th International Congress of ORL and I wrote to you. I don't know if you got the letter, but I drank Tokay to your health—it is something anyway.

In September, though I am not a cardiology patient I had an emergency operation caused by a misbehaving prostate. After a short hospital stay, I resumed my activities, still doing surgery. But this year again in September an adenoma in the right colon did bother me, so I went back on the operating table. I am happy to have now a good diagnosis about the adenoma's origin and metastasis. My convalescence was rapid and I recovered very well, hungry all the time . . . not having any more colon problems . . . So I go on, organizing an international colloquium in Hanoi on nasopharyngeal cancer. I was expecting Dr. Yves Cachin to come here but he has cardiac problems, therefore I had to go to Paris to confer with him and the others from the Health Ministry. The trip was long: I am going to Hanoi via Hong Kong, New Delhi and Karachi. We have to be at Charles de Gaulle airport in Paris at 6 a.m.

On our way to Paris with my assistant, we wanted to stay in New Delhi. We had to get in a bus to Air India and finally arrived at 10 am Paris time, with no rest—Paris has changed: too many people, too much noise and the cost of living went up, alas! I will stay a few weeks depending on my workload. There were conferences lasting over five hours, but it is all right, I take it well for my age. As I am used to getting up very early, to do calisthenics, I use the few moments of relaxation to write you and ask about you: will you come to spend Christmas in Paris? Anyway, I think I can write you from Paris directly, and I hope to get a note from you very soon.

Goodbye, Jacqueline, Merry Christmas and a Happy New Year for 1983. In 1983 we plan to come to Europe, then I will give lectures in Algeria and then my daughter returns to her studies at Gustave Roussy, and it will be good to meet with you! Who knows!

Very affectionately,
Tran Hu Tuoc

X

Nostalgia

Jacqueline had some critical thoughts upon re-reading the letters from Tuoc. Tuoc had gotten married but never mentioned it, and at seventy years of age had a son that was sixteen and a daughter, that was twenty-two and was studying medicine. He had only mentioned one child when he talked about adopting a tiny girl! He never talked about marrying and his family life! He had affairs in Paris while they were engaged . . . his affective life was his own! If Jacqueline had married Tuoc, she would only have been a helper to his work, always in the background, and could never have achieved any scientific research on her own. Another thing that came to mind was that any kind of dependence of one country by another is harmful to creativity . . . while the colonies were given all the social benefits of France, and there are many, this did not make up for the inequality between the French and the Vietnamese, which was based on French colonial domination, greed and racism.

Jacqueline concluded that she had made the right choice in refusing to go to Vietnam or even to marry Tuoc and enjoy a life of plenty in Paris with the company of a frustrated man. No professional success, she believed, could have overcome Tuoc's patriotism and devotion to his ancient civilization.

In conclusion, Jacqueline believes she made the right choices all along and knows that her life was full of all kinds of experiences and challenges, and she is now very much at peace with her past, and her losses. She is happy to know that Tuoc has two successful children, a girl studying to be a physician and a boy reaching for Les Grandes Ecoles. In Houston, Jacqueline has many wonderful friends, old and young, including her niece and nephew, and her lovely young Mexican friend and her husband. Telephone chats with Simone have also filled the void of not having her own children. Her older friends all have their own problems and families, but they keep in touch regularly. She keeps in close telephone contact with the distant ones: Louise, Rosa, and Renée. Each day Jacqueline feels so lucky to live in a lovely, warm house in a peaceful country, to exercise daily in her outdoor pool and hot tub in the landscaped backyard, to have help in keeping the house and lovely garden, and to have enough financial security that she has nothing to worry about until death occurs, perhaps in her sleep! If she had made the choice to wear a star during the Nazi era in Paris, she would have missed all her past, and instead she would have fed the weeds in the dump where she would have rotted! Her last choice is to give her body to the Medical School and have it incinerated anonymously, in memory.

After retiring, Jacqueline had the opportunity to return to her first love: painting. She has become very materialistic; she enjoys beautiful objects, and clothing. She became a gourmet and a wine lover. When she reads letters that were written by the two most important men in her life, she feels that all their dreams were exclusively in their minds, and that their image of her was completely false. Finally, Jacqueline believes that her medical research has indirectly improved the care of patients with spinal cord injury. She also thinks that her lifelike paintings give her friends some pleasure! She is so thankful to have the affection of Ann, Alain, Elisabeth and Jean Francois, as well as many other wonderful friends. Her recent loss of Simone was difficult. Like when Bob died, she felt abandoned! But Simone was four months short of ninety, and there has to be an end to life. Now Jacqueline is waiting for her turn. She loves her care-taker, Dr. Kim Bloom, and his wife, Robin. At home she has help from a kind lady, although she is frustrated because they cannot chat. Elva speaks only Spanish and Jacqueline never learned! She also has the help of an old Mexican gardener. She was lucky to have been helped in renovating her house by the son of Evalina, a doctor friend she met at TIRR. She enjoys the friendly help of MT, who, with Elisabeth, helps her with her health problems, taking her to the physicians' offices in the Medical Center, and keeping her company when she is hospitalized at Methodist Hospital. Throughout Jacqueline's professional life, Betty Kilday helped her publish readable arti-cles using her knowledge of English. Now Betty helps with the story of Jacqueline's life. Bill still helps her maintain the lovely fountain he built for her, and takes her to events connected with the Houston Museum of Fine Art. And to this day, she enjoys the Houston Ballet with Elisabeth. She has had much to enjoy, instead of rotting in the earth of a concentration camp in Germany.

The main shadow in Jacqueline's life is the absence of Simone. She was hoping to have her read her memoirs in a critical manner, hoping to spend hours discussing opinions about events that they shared . . . no one else can do it, neither Rosa or Louise, because they shared only a small part of Jacque-line's life.

So Jacqueline has only her memory and a few letters to help here reconstruct the past. Therefore her story is biased! She has tried to be honest and faithful to facts . . . but this is only possible to a point!